Communicating as a Mental Health Carer

Paul Bonham
RMN RNT BA MA MEd

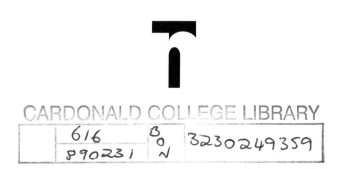

Published in 2004 by:
Nelson Thornes Ltd
Delta Place
27 Bath Road
CHELTENHAM
GL53 7TH
United Kingdom

05 06 07 / 10 9 8 7 6 5 4 3 2

A catalogue record for this book is available from the British Library

ISBN 0 7487 7291 X

Page make-up by Acorn Bookwork, Salisbury, Wiltshire

Printed in Great Britain by Ashford Colour Press

Contents

PREFACE

This book is primarily aimed at student nurses, who are just about to go on, or who are part-way through, a clinical placement. It can also be usefully read by anyone who regularly works in mental health settings. An assumption made throughout this book is that many early placements for student mental health nurses are likely to be in institutional settings, i.e. wards or day hospitals. Therefore some scenarios take place in those settings while others take place in a community setting. The rudimentary skills in this book are intended to help beginners in these situations, even the situation where the student is told to 'Go and talk to the patients'. (It still happens, I am regularly told by students themselves.) Parts of the book are aimed at the period where the student may feel a little more comfortable in the placement. Maybe they have started to get to know a small number of the patients. Other sections may be of interest to more experienced students, and even qualified nurses. All the skills and techniques described work, in terms of contributing something useful to patient/client care. They have all been tried with patients, clients, colleagues, relatives and students, sometimes accidentally at first, but then on purpose.

The reason for this book is that one of the many problems facing student nurses (and to some extent more experienced practitioners) is knowing where and how to start when faced with the ever expanding body of professional literature and, sometimes, over-inclusive module reading lists. No textbook or curriculum has ever provided comfortable certainties about the 'right thing to do' when meeting the needs of people who are experiencing the distress caused by mental illness. Discussion continues about the relative merits of different approaches to care which are often perceived as competing ideologies by 'warring professionals' (Egan 2002). This book is intended as a practical guide to a selection of some (not all) commonly encountered situations in mental health nursing. In it are attempts to provide some ideas for beginners as to how to manage (rather than cope) in these situations.

The contents should guide the reader to the part needed. This could be when anticipating a professional interaction, during one (some conversations can last the course of a shift, on and off), or when thinking and reflecting afterwards about how it went.

The book does not claim to be comprehensive in scope as the target reader is the 'beginner', but it does aim to be comprehensively introductory. It attempts to identify and illustrate the skills, techniques and ideas that are often transferable between different situations, as well as the skills that are more specific. Clinically experienced readers will notice that no attempt is made to offer any kind of linear structure or framework to the interventions described. It was felt, from the author's own personal experience, that at the stage of the beginner it is sometimes very difficult to be thinking of what to say at all to the person in front of you, never mind trying to apply some theoretical framework to the inter-vention. The beginner's attempts at professional interventions are often largely based on their spontaneous responses to people. The skills, techniques and ideas described can be used in such a way. They are intended to add to, or enhance, the beginner's repertoire of possibilities. However, many of the skills, techniques and ideas have their roots in the works, ideas and philosophies of Carl Rogers – the Person Centred or Humanistic Approach (Rogers 1951), Gerard Egan – the Three Stage Helping Process (Egan 2002), and John Heron – the concept of having a clear range of 'Intentions' (Heron 2001). The reason for the choice of Rogers' approach was because this seems to have a very wide application and can at least be *attempted* by most people in many situations. Egan was chosen because many people who look for professional mental health care are experiencing, or experience, difficulties in coping with life problems. Sometimes these people can be helped to find their own answers by the guided use of a problem solving approach. The Egan framework is described by McLeod (1998, p. 213) as 'intensely practical and pragmatic'. This makes it attractive to some patients and some carers who prefer such a way of working. Heron's approach is also chosen because it is a useful framework to attempt to bring order and focus to the often unfocussed, chaotic world of the beginner.

The content is not intended to be used as a guide to therapy but as a way of starting and sustaining a rapport and broadening the beginner's communication skills. If appropriate, the use of frameworks and a more structured way of working can be usefully incorporated into the experienced carer's way of working.

At many points in the text you will see that there are also sections titled 'Discussion points'. The intention here is that these can be used during classroom sessions by teachers. They can also be used to develop the themes that are raised in the text, by the student reader themselves, especially if they are studying a curriculum that uses enquiry-based learning as one of the teaching approaches. The sometimes extreme viewpoints expressed in these sections are not necessarily reflective of the author's opinion. They are intended to promote thinking and debate around the issues raised, and are sometimes deliberately naïve.

It is also important to note that currently there seems to be a feeling of increasing dissatisfaction and uneasiness with mental health services in Britain: 'that in the main rely on coercion and medication rather than engaging with the people who receive [the services]' (Laurance 2002, p. 4). Commentators in the media, service users and some mental health professionals (Johnstone 2000) are critical both of the face-to-face service provided by professionals and the philosophy driving governmental changes. In addition, the stigma attached to mental illness shows no sign of abating in this new millennium: 'an age which sees people with mental health problems as dangerous and unpredictable' (Muijen 1996, cited in Hopkins and Walsey 2002, p. 21).

It is against this uneasy background that this book is offered.

Throughout this text the term 'patient' is used, with the rationale that this word best represents the situation of the person in institutional care. 'Client' will be used to describe the person in any other setting. This is done in the awareness that other terms such as 'service user' are preferred by some.

Also you will note that the carer is often referred to as a 'nurse'. There are two reasons for this. Firstly, nurses of all grades are the largest occupational group in mental health caring. Secondly, this book is aimed directly at the experience of the student nurse undertaking the current 'Making a Difference' curriculum. However, the skills and situations described and explained have relevance for many other mental health carers.

None of the skills, techniques or ideas should be tried without discussing them first with your assessor or mentor to check that they will be appropriate for the situation. In some instances a useful learning technique might be to talk it through or role-play it with your mentor.

In a few examples of dialogue, swear words are used. The intention is to provide examples that are real. Patients and clients sometimes use 'bad language', as people do in our wider society. Often this is directed at their professional carers. They do this for many reasons. It can signal distress. They may be trying to make a point. It may be part of their culture and they may not be aware that it might cause offence. Whatever the reason, it is the job of the effective mental health nurse to make constructive use of the material provided by the patient. This might mean asking the patient to temper their language, reflecting back the content and/or feeling of what they have just said, or even incorporating some of the same language into the professional response. Whatever the reason, the nurse has to consider how to manage this situation. Some possible answers to this dilemma are in this book. I felt that the inclusion of this material was important for several reasons:

- It is realistic. Some patients/ clients use strong language for a range of reasons, just like anyone else
- It is important that nurses think about how to respond to strong language in a positive way
- It is important that nurses know how to make sense of the emotions that sometimes accompany strong language, to help the patient
- The inclusion of this material in this book gives the student an opportunity to think through/discuss how they might react in similar situations, as they will *definitely* occur.

Many of the references used to support interventions are sourced from recent journals. Many of the references used to support descriptions of disorders are from textbooks. This is a deliberate strategy as most of the information regarding disorders has not changed very recently whereas the use of journals was thought to best capture contemporary clinical thinking and practice.

It is hoped that any reader of this book will be able to detect an empathy for what it is like to be a student mental health nurse, a qualified mental health nurse, a mental health teacher, a patient, and a relative of the latter. The author, is, or has been, very close to all of these roles.

Throughout this book, all names used and scenarios described are invented by the author and entirely fictitious.

HOW TO USE THIS BOOK

The first section sets the scene, primarily for the student nurse, although again, newcomers to mental health care may find this useful. A range of clinical settings is described, as are some of the different approaches used by contemporary mental health professionals. Clarification of what the student role involves is attempted, as is an addressing of some of the challenges that most students have to face.

The skills, techniques and ideas throughout the book are illustrated by examples of dialogue. Some examples are brief and others are extensive. They are all useable by students, once the basic principles, described and explained in Chapters 1–3 are understood. In relation to the current 'Making a Difference' nursing curriculum, these three parts are sequenced deliberately. Chapter 1 describes skills that would be useable, or could be attempted by, most first year students from *any* speciality (not just mental health) in *any* mental health setting. Chapter 2 skills could be useable, or may be attempted by, most second-year mental health students and Chapter 3 skills by most third-year mental health students (these groups are not meant to be prescriptive – they are suggestions only). All are preceded, followed or interspersed with explanatory rationale and discussion of the 'pros and cons' of particular verbal and non-verbal interventions. It is not the intention to present an idealised account of practice, but a fairly easy to understand portrayal of the reality of day-to-day mental health interventions with a continuing intention to care and help (Heron 2001).

As mentioned above, the examples throughout the book are not meant to be prescriptive of what must, or should be said, in a particular situation. They are suggestions as to what might, or could be said to achieve a specific outcome or range of outcomes or intentions. As such, they are intended to be read critically. The outcomes described will, of course, not be the only ones possible. People who are seriously distressed, and sometimes seriously disturbed, are not always welcoming of carers' endeavours to be therapeutic or consoling. Many patients are resistive of carers' efforts at helpful interventions. That does not mean our efforts are in vain.

Coping with suspiciousness, indifference, or outright hostility from patients and clients is a difficult but necessary part of our professional role. Cautious, or sometimes assertive, persistence may often eventually result in a degree at least of acceptance, rapport and sometimes even trust, which may be helpful enough. We should also not forget that many users of statutory mental health services view themselves as psychiatric survivors (Thomas *et al* 1997, Wright and Giddey 1993, Johnstone 2000, Laurance 2003, Barker 1999) or combatants, not just of their illness or disorder but also of the system that claims to be treating and caring for them, i.e. the nurses, doctors and other professionals involved. Passive compliance is convenient for us but is not always a sign of positive mental health in the patient.

In Chapters 4 and 5, a range of stories and scenarios from both the perspective of the nurse, the person being cared for, and their family and significant others is presented. The person-centred approach (Rogers 1951) is used, or at least, inferred throughout the book, together with the more contemporary spirits of collaboration (Hopkins and Walsey 2002, Egan 2002, McLeod 1998, Barker 1999), patient empowerment (Fitzimons 2002), and autonomy (McLeod 1998) that are the goals and ideals of many mental health carers trying to resist the pull of the medical model (Evans 1995).

Chapter 6 refocuses on the reader and how some of the skills from Chapters 1–3 can be used to manage actually doing the job, given that, at the time of writing, nurses of all specialities are leaving their career in worryingly large numbers and many students consider doing this even before they qualify (RCN 2003).

Suggestions for further reading reflect the author's own diverse preferences and prejudices, The writers that students and colleagues have consistently found the most helpful are also identified.

ACKNOWLEDGEMENTS

Thanks to Rod Bell for suggesting a book in the first place and to Dr Paul Crawford for encouragement and advice in making this a reality. Both colleagues provided generous editorial advice and further suggestions.

Thanks to Helen Broadfield, Eve Thould and Chris Wortley at Nelson Thornes for helping me through this process for the first time.

For further content suggestions and corrections, thanks to: Lillian Canning, Ann Edwards, Lesley Legg, Sam Murray, Graham Peden, and Sefton Redshaw; for IT and library support, Neil Buxton and Dianne Winter.

Also very special thanks to Polly Sealey and Mrs Joan Robinson for much encouragement and support

Paul Bonham

To my daughters, Soeli and Thea

In memory of the late Theresa Duffy

Introduction: setting the scene

Mental health care settings

This section will describe and review some of the different care settings that mental health student carers are likely to encounter.

Older adult – organic

This setting involves caring for people who are suffering primarily from a disintegration of brain physiology and thus of brain function. In the latter stages of the disorder, this often presents as a change of personality. An early sign is the gradual disappearance of short-term memory where events that happened many years ago can still be recalled (Thomas *et al.* 1997). Unfortunately, sufferers seem to become vulnerable to physical illness as well (Olds 1995), especially in institutional settings. The student working in this type of placement will have experience of communicating helpfully not only with the patients but also with the relatives. The relatives may be distressed at the double loss they are experiencing (Moyle 2002), or they may even be relieved that the weight of responsibility of day-to-day care has been taken from them. The student will be exposed to a range of cognitive (thought and perception) disorders that are untypical of most other settings. The responses and reaction of the sufferers to usual human interactions will be very different. This, combined with the management of physical illness and the difficulties of significant others makes for a rich, but tiring and demanding, learning environment/experience.

Discussion point

How does the mental health carer come to terms with the fact that at the present time the process of disintegration can only be possibly slowed down by a combination of medication and interpersonal interventions? It cannot be reversed. There is no cure.

Older adult – functional

This term describes a group of people (usually over 65 years of age) who are suffering with similar types of mental health difficulties to younger people. They may be suffering from depressive illness, psychosis, bipolar disorder, and so on. The fact that an older person is experiencing mental disorder may have a different impact on themselves and their relatives from the suffering of a younger person. For example, the stresses of a manic episode may be considerably worsened because of the increased physical fragility of a person compared with when they were younger, especially, for example, with regard to falling (Norman and Redfern 1997). The learning experience will be enriched when the student becomes aware of the impact, on the relatives and significant others, of functional disorders on older adults.

Day hospital

The experience here will be that of helping to treat people of all ages, but most often older adults, who can manage with professional support during the day. They will cope over the weekend and overnight, either with informal carers or sometimes on their own. The treatments offered in these settings range from social groups through to one-to-one counselling sessions, depending on the assessed needs of the person. Daily contact or planned contact on a regular basis means that interventions from other agencies such as community psychiatric nurses (CPNs – sometimes also known as community mental health nurses, CMHNs) or re-admission can be arranged quickly if, and when, relapse starts to occur. These settings therefore have a very useful assessment and monitoring, as well as treatment, function.

Rehabilitation

Community-based

These settings often carry out the function of acting as a 'halfway house' for people who are ready to leave the 24-hour type of institutional care but are assessed as still needing some professional support. Some of the therapeutic strategies and treatments the student might expect to see would involve continuing assessment and monitoring of social functioning – e.g. how people behave in group or social settings such as a pub or supermarket. The person's ability to manage day-to-day living in a more isolated setting than the institution would also be assessed. For example the person could be housed in a flat or house and regularly supported and monitored to see if and how they manage in this situation.

Institution-based

Of necessity, this may involve patients living in close proximity to other patients, although people receiving care in this setting usually have their own personal space. In many ways the aims of care are the same as those of the community-based setting described above. The person in care is further from independent community living, though, in terms of their ability to manage. They are likely to be seen as needing closer monitoring and a more protected or supported lifestyle.

The time-span of this could be months or much longer-term (Varcarolis 1998). The experience of the student could be similar to the community setting, in terms of seeing how the patient manages in a range of different situations. The student will also have the opportunity (under supervision) to monitor prescribed medication, model appropriate social behaviours both in and outside the institution and, importantly, at all times try to reduce the patient's reliance on institutional support.

Community Mental Health Team

This is likely to take several forms. Community Mental Health Teams (CMHTs) tend to have caseloads that specialise in certain age groups. The student experience will therefore be focused around the needs of older adults, adults in a continuing care situation or adults in an acute situation. The student will become more aware of the differences in the relationships between a range of professional carers and clients when the latter are on their own territory. The student will become aware that the majority of people needing professional mental health support in settings like this are much closer to primary care (Gillam 2002) than the secondary care that was predominant as recently as 20 years ago. This care setting will be highly conducive to the student witnessing the development, sustaining and termination of therapeutic relationships. This is much more difficult to see and do in the often more repressive atmosphere of institutional care (Laurance, 2003).

Acute adult setting

This care setting caters generally for ages from mid-teenage to the sixties and has a group of patients with a wide range of problems. All people admitted are individually assessed. A care plan agreed with the patient is implemented whenever appropriate, although this is sometimes difficult, given the state of mind of some people on admission. Often a significant percentage of people who are treated in this environment are being detained under sections of the Mental Health Act (1983). Similarly many people admitted to these areas are seen as being a danger to themselves or perhaps others (Barker 2003). The range of disorders could include people with depressive illnesses, psychoses, substance abuse detoxification, episodic self-harm, bipolar disorder, personality disorder (depending on the local willingness to treat), and people who suffer from complex disorders and seem to be dispossessed and lost in our society: 'The reality for many people with mental health problems is that, apart from professionals and other service users, they have no friends or community' (Bates 2002, p. 21).

Some of the acute settings are mixed-sex. At the time of writing, this is being addressed (Firn 1995, cited in Thomas *et al.* 1997, and others) in terms of returning to the situation of around 20 years ago, when the sexes were not usually mixed.

Specialist areas

Assertive outreach

These teams, based in the community, were originally set up to address the continuing difficulties of the severely and enduring mentally ill (Libberton 2000). Many clients are likely to be 'unreceptive or positively hostile to service interventions ... usually living on the margins of society ... and have become disenfranchised from the services to which they are entitled' (Williamson 2003, pp. 24–25). The student experience is likely to include seeing team members with necessarily limited caseloads, a truly multidisciplinary approach using a wide range of intervention skills. Team members may also visit clients in their own homes, working in pairs to reduce risk whenever appropriate. The difficulties of engaging meaningfully will be clearly seen, and how the professional handles this struggle can be discussed: 'Clients may engage and disengage, accept and reject interventions for no apparent reason. This can feel confusing and frustrating' (Williamson 2003, p. 25).

Crisis resolution/intervention
The rationale of this team is to respond quickly to mental health crisis. A philosophy used as the foundation of these teams is: 'A crisis was not an unfortunate event that had to be defused as quickly as possible by removing the supposedly sick person, rather, it was a unique opportunity to do vital therapeutic work, as tensions that might be dormant and hidden for years erupted into the open' (Johnstone 2000, p. 94).

One of the primary aims of this kind of team is to try to prevent or at least delay admission to hospital by treating a person in their own environment.

Secure/forensic
The student will experience the strategies that are used to try to help and rehabilitate some of the most damaged, distressed and distressing of the people who are users of professional mental health care. The care setting will necessarily be medium- to high-security involving almost inevitably a locked care environment. There will be more emphasis on security devices such as closed-circuit television (CCTV) and personal alarms (Beer *et al.* 2001). Staffing levels reflect the continuing risk to carers who work in this environment. The institutional and personal philosophy of carers who work in forensic settings is sometimes different from those who work, for example, in community, acute, and older person teams. Part of the student experience involves coming to terms with these differences and making sense of where, in this culture, the student 'fits'.

Discussion point

How do mental health carers working in this type of environment create and sustain therapeutic relationships? Do they ever manage to achieve this? If so, what might be the evidence that they have reached this quality of interaction with their patient(s)? What is the point, given that most of these patients will probably remain in or around institutional care for the rest of their lives?

Substance abuse/misuse
As with the secure/forensic experience, a significant part of the learning experience for the student in this setting is to consider the similarities and differences in philosophy and attitudes between carers who work with this group of service users and carers who work with other groups. The needs and drives of the

users/clients of this service will be quite different in many respects from other groups. The difficulties of creating and sustaining the therapeutic relationship are also probably in some respects quite different (Tober 1994; see also sections 4.6 and 5.7).

Discussion point

Given that substance abuse is increasing on a worldwide scale, what can individual Substance Abuse health-care workers achieve with the clients on their case loads? How do they come to terms with the reality that some of their clients will die or will never recover? How do they manage the constantly increasing number of referrals? What responses are coming from other services who also feel the impact of this demographic and societal change, such as acute services, forensic and Child and Family services?

Child and family

Here the focus of care is also widened to include other family members and not just the child. Referrals are likely to come from a much wider range of individuals, such as the child's parent, teacher, school nurse or social worker. The relationships between the family members, the history of the family and the patterns of behaviour or 'scripts' (Altschuler 1997) are all considered by the carer, who often will take an integrative approach when trying to help the child. Again a very useful exercise for the student is to try to distil which approaches would be useful for them in their future practice.

Discussion point

Do children referred to this service often carry on being referred in their adult life? What could be the differences between those who are and those who aren't? How do carers who work in this service create therapeutic relationships with children? What are the differences between these and therapeutic relationships with adults? How do they avoid stigmatising their users/clients?

Behaviour Therapy Unit

There is likely to be less time spent investing in the therapeutic relationship, compared to most other approaches: 'Some have suggested that clients can be treated with a self-help manual' (Ghosh 1988, cited in Thomas *et al.* 1997, p. 461), and more time spent addressing the immediate problems experienced by the user. This is a very pragmatic approach to mental health care. Unlike the approach in Child and Family it is less likely that the history and relationships of the user will be explored in much depth. The approach is very 'here and now' (Nelson Jones 2002) and based on well-established problem-solving principles and the belief that anything learned can be unlearned (Thomas *et al.* 1997). As before, it is interesting for the student to observe the assessment techniques used by the practitioners and also again try to make sense of the attitudes and philosophies that drive the carers who use these techniques.

Discussion point

Would more time invested in the creation of a therapeutic relationship with clients who use this service help or hinder the progress of treatments? If this approach works with so little time spent creating a therapeutic relationship, why do we bother doing this in other services?

Psychodynamic Psychotherapy Unit

The chances of students experiencing very much of this therapeutic approach in its purest sense are very restricted because of the nature of the care setting, which is highly controlled and contracted (the clients are very clear about boundaries and the limitations of the treatment offered and they agree to be bound by these). The relationship between the carer and user is very exclusive and does not naturally lend itself to any observation opportunities, apart from circumstances of co-working or supervision. A large part of the work is helping the client understand, or come to terms with, events and relationships from the past, especially parental. This is then used to help them become aware of the impact of these on their life as it is now. Part of this process involves the influence of the relationship between the client and the carer in terms of the 'transferences' (Nelson Jones 1997, Bloye and Davies 1999) and the learning from this that can be used to help the patient. This is another reason why this mental health setting does not lend itself easily to student experience, apart from people who are students only of the psychodynamic psychotherapeutic approach.

Discussion point

Given that this is a very expensive treatment approach and that its evidence base is much smaller than those of approaches such as cognitive behaviour therapy (Gumley et al. 2003, Turkington 2002, Oei 1999) what is the justification for its continuance as a specialist service, rather than being used as another tool of the eclectic or integrative mental health worker?

Self-harm liaison

As above, opportunities for direct student contact are limited because of the nature of the work carried out in this type of placement. Clients seen in these circumstances are, with few exceptions, especially vulnerable and sensitive. It is essential that the carer develops a trusting relationship very quickly. The presence of a third party could impair that process; however the student experience, when it arises in this working environment, is likely to be very valuable in terms of exposure to assessment and referral skills.

Discussion point

How do carers working with this client group come to terms with the fact that they are always assessing and are never part of the implementation of nursing care? How do they manage to create a therapeutic relationship so quickly? What is their evidence that one exists? Is such a relationship feasible at all, in the short time that they have with their clients?

Court diversion/criminal justice liaison

As above, the main aim within this area of clinical work is to provide a screening service. People who have apparently committed a criminal offence are assessed while in custody: 'A pivotal role can be played by CPNs in diversion, thereby alleviating the tremendous personal distress experienced by mentally ill people who become caught up in the criminal justice system' (Hillis 1993, cited by Thomas *et al.* 1997, p. 118). The aim of the assessment, and sometimes subsequent referral, is to ensure, as much as is humanly possible, that people who are influenced by mental illness to commit an offence receive appropriate help rather than being processed through the court system: 'The results of such assessments can play an essential role in informing the court's decision on disposal of an individual' (Thomas *et al.* 1997, p. 118).

Discussion point

What are the characteristics of the creation of a therapeutic relationship with people in this situation? How is a rapport created under such difficult conditions in the time available and considering the environment in which the assessments are carried out?

Challenging behaviour

Many people who suffer with mental health problems present with challenging behaviour in terms of the difficulties they present to people who live and work around them and the people who try to care for them. This is true both in informal and professional care settings. The term 'challenging behaviour', when applied to people who are being looked after in professional settings, is generally understood to mean that they cannot be managed in some private sector care settings, such as nursing homes and sheltered housing, because of the extreme nature of their behaviour. Or, their behaviour presents such difficulties for their carers, outside of a relatively controlled setting, that they need to be cared for in a more specialised environment: 'Acute disturbance can also become chronic disturbance' (Beer *et al.* 2001, p. 14).

Some patients who might be considered to need this type of more concentrated care are those who are not only suffering from long-term and chronic mental health difficulties but have also become even more disabled by the influence of many years of psychiatric containment in institutions (Laurance 2003, p. 20). The combination of these two aspects often results in behaviours that are difficult to manage: 'Many of the patients in this group act in such a way as to tax the understanding of the team (Beer *et al.* 2001, p. 109). They can also be very resistant to any type of therapeutic approach that might otherwise produce or encourage some evidence of a therapeutic result.

Discussion point

How do carers in this environment remain optimistic when many of the people they are caring for are likely to remain in care for their entire lives, and any improvement as a result of treatment is likely to be very small and transient?

APPROACHES TO DELIVERY OF MENTAL HEALTH CARE

There are many ways to help and treat people who are suffering from mental health disorders. Most of the mainstream methods are covered below. (Some of the material in the section above is replicated necessarily here.) In every placement the student carer will see one, or a combination of these approaches being used.

Medical/physical

This is probably the most traditional approach, with the longest history in our society. Much of the history of psychiatry/mental health care in the Western world is based on this model (Thomas *et al.* 1997). In many clinical areas it is still probably the primary approach. This term is usually taken to mean approaches such as the use of medication, electroconvulsive therapy (ECT) and attention to the more physical aspects of the human condition such as sleep, mobility, nutrition, elimination and so on. Often a model such as Roper, Logan and Tierney's Activities of Living (Roper *et al.* 2000) would be used to assess within this approach.

One benefit to clients is that treatments can be easily explained, in that symptoms are identified and treated. The same benefit applies to the carers. The student will experience seeing the client treated in this type of placement using an approach that places a great reliance on the use of physical (somatic) therapies. Some contemporary writers and practitioners question the effectiveness of this approach because deeper issues are not addressed, such as spirituality (Thompson 2000, Warner and Nicholls 2000) and gender: 'What most women with psychiatric diagnoses need is, first, to be helped to see that they are only part of the problem, and second, to get angry enough about it to make some real changes. The medical model cannot allow for this' (Johnstone 2000, p. 119). Gelder *et al.* (1999, p. 58) suggest: 'It is less useful ... in the study of neuroses and personality disorders'. The medical model does, however, seem to be the leading approach in the West: 'Much of modern psychiatric care is dominated by the medical model' (Thomas *et al.* 1997, p. 27).

Discussion point

Why is there so much criticism of this approach when it makes so much sense? What could be more logical than: 'diagnosis, treatment and cure' (Crepaz-Kreay 2003)? Isn't it logical to treat the symptoms and not take account of any possible underlying factors?

Cognitive Behavioural Therapy (CBT)

This is a very versatile approach in terms of its flexibility and ability to be used with a wide range of clients in many settings by a wide range of carers (Gelder *et al.* 1999). A reason why this approach is more patient/client-friendly is the capacity for it to be used not only one-to-one but with groups and in community, day hospital and institutional settings. There is an investment in the establishment of the therapeutic relationship and exploration of the way the person sees their world. McLeod (1998, p. 62) describes it as a 'change focused approach [that pays] close attention to the cognitive processes through which people monitor and control their behaviour'. The person's perceptions are compared with the objective evidence that supports their subjective reality. The aim of this style of therapy is to establish a more positive approach that can be used realistically by that person. It does need active participation and involvement on the part of the patient or client to be effective, like many other therapeutic approaches. The experience for the student will be that of being exposed to an approach that can be used in almost any setting and that has a substantial weight of evidence suggesting that it is effective (Abramowitz 2001, Christensen 2003, Embling 2002).

Discussion point

If this approach makes so much sense, is so effective and is useable by such a wide range of professionals in such a wide range of situations, how is it that there doesn't seem to be much evidence of any major impact on the number of depressed people and suicides in the Western world? Barker (1992 cited in Barker 1999, p. 154) suggests: 'By the year 2020, major clinical depression will be the second most important burden of disease in the world. Truly we have entered a new age of melancholy.'

Psychodynamic

This is an approach whose aim is to help clients make sense of their early relationships and the impact these have on the way they are now. This can be integrated into other approaches but in its purest form it is carried out by specially trained practitioners in a contracted environment with well-defined boundaries. The relationship between the therapist and the client is also examined in terms of its use as a metaphor for the client's past, present and future relationships with others (Gelder *et al.* 1999).

Discussion point

How does it help the client when they come to understand why they behave/think the way they do? What happens next? Why is it so difficult to provide hard evidence that this approach actually works in the same way that the cognitive behavioural approach is apparently proven (Gumley *et al.* 2003, Turkington 2002, Oei 1999).

Psychosocial

This approach takes an optimistic view of the patient/client and focuses on their strengths: 'encourage and foster responsibility for putting these abilities into action, rather than assuming the patient to be ill' (Beer *et al.* 2001, p. 128). In this sense it is likely to be combined with another approach, or will be a combination of several approaches (Altschuler 1997), as its intention is to empower rather than pathologise. Johnstone (2000, p. 35) suggests that this approach is 'a model which sees psychiatric breakdown as resulting from a mixture of psychological factors (mainly past and present relationship difficulties, and sometimes a spiritual crisis of values and beliefs), often accompanied by social and financial problems'. 'The client's difficulties in living are revealed, contained and explored in the daily life of the community and a newly emergent self is nurtured' (Watkins 2001, p. 151; see also Bradshaw 2000).

Socialisation

Again, this is often carried out as part of a wider integrated or eclectic approach and is based on the premise that we are social beings and cannot live healthily in isolation (Norman and Redfern 1997). This approach will involve the client going into social situations that previously might contribute to their difficulties. While in these social situations the client is assessed, supported and treated by a member of the care team. This particular approach lends itself well to being carried out by supervised students, who get the chance to create a level of relationship that helps the client to trust not only the student but also their ability to carry out the therapy. A significant part of the carer's role both in this and the behavioural approach (described below) is to support the client while they are being 'desensitised' in the environment that is difficult for them (Barry 1998, p. 367).

Discussion point

Is this an example of how mental health services often pathologise something that is part of our normal life? A contemporary example might be the labelling of difficult people who don't fit into easily definable diagnostic categories as 'borderline personality disorder' (Bloye and Davies 1999).

Behavioural

As above but often with a more specific focus. This approach can be used to effectively treat people who are suffering with phobic conditions, post-traumatic stress disorder (PTSD; Newell and Gournay 2000) and many other conditions that restrict the person's lifestyle. A common example is the condition known as agoraphobia (fear of being alone in open or public places where escape might be difficult; Varcarolis 2000). A way of helping someone whose life is disrupted by this phobia would be to take them gradually into the very environment that is troubling them. The usual experience is that, after initially raised anxiety, the levels of anxiety gradually drop to the point that the person treated in this way is able to confront the situation on their own, or with less intensive support. This approach seems to require less emphasis on the development of a therapeutic relationship compared to, for instance, the cognitive approach, which values this aspect highly: 'Behaviour modification does not sit easily within a counselling relationship' (McLeod 1998, p. 67) (see also Cognitive behavioural approach).

Discussion point

If this approach is so distanced from any attempt to create a therapeutic relationship, can't it be carried out by people who are not particularly caring? If it is so simple to do, why don't less highly trained people carry it out or give the clients an instruction manual (Ghosh 1988, cited in Thomas et al. 1997).

Humanistic

This is another approach that has wide potential for many situations, settings and clients. Often attributed to Carl Rogers (Rogers 1951), this consists of a cluster of human characteristics that Rogers suggested facilitate helping and therapeutic relationships with people. He proposed and practised an empathic, non-judgemental and accepting approach. These qualities, with a non-directive manner, he suggested, would help many people to help themselves, using their own inherent drives towards the positive.

Deceptively simple in its concept, this approach is actually much more difficult to use in its purest sense than the description suggests. However, as with many other approaches it can often be used as one component of a range of techniques available to the creative mental health carer.

Discussion point

Rogers apparently viewed the human race as inherently good: 'his underlying assumption was that each person carried a universal morality, and would have a bodily sense of what was right or wrong in any situation' (McLeod 1988 p. 95). This belief was a cornerstone of his philosophy of care. How can this be true given the constant human conflict in the world? For further reading around this subject, see Thorne (2002).

Eclectic

This is used by probably the great majority of mental health carers, especially when they first start working clinically. The term describes the attempt to help the person in front of you, using whatever comes to mind at the time and based on their needs and your skill level, or 'drawing from different theories in response to the demands of practice' (Nelson Jones 1997, p. 7). It is driven by the desire to help but can be based on a more intuitive and sometimes less organised approach or use of technique, with the focus being the perceived needs of the recipient. Lazarus (cited in Nelson Jones 1997) suggested that there were two types of eclectics, systematic and unsystematic. Whatever the academic description, this method continues to be used by many nurses and can be very effective, when used by the thoughtful nurse, as it is so patient/client-focused.

Discussion point

Isn't this just a complicated term for 'making it up as you go along'? If we do this, what do we need training for?

Integrative

This approach is more planned, coherent and thoughtful and less chaotic than the previous one. The carer who uses an integrative approach will deliberately combine a number of different models and philosophies to fit what they see as the needs of the person in front of them. Their approach can change over time as the needs of their client changes so it has a very strong organic sense about it. McLeod (1998) calls it 'harmonious'.

A contemporary example of an effective integrative approach is the widening use of Cognitive Behavioural Therapy – a combination of both cognitive and behavioural principles.

Discussion point

How can this possibly be effective as an approach when you never really know what the client is going to say or do next? People are unpredictable aren't they?

Issues around the role of the student

Established members of any clinical team would have certain expectations of any student working with them for a period of a few weeks or months. The relationship is necessarily two-way.

Expectations of the placement team members

The team is very likely to be multidisciplinary or multispeciality.

- *The student is reliable.* You turn up on time in the right place. Team members and assessors/mentors do not like the distraction of wondering where you are and, if they don't know, should they be doing anything about it? Should they be waiting in case you turn up? Do they need to let your school base know? Should they be recording your absence in an objectives book? Should they be trying to contact you at home? If you are stuck/ill/late, let them know.
- *The student is presentable.* You look appropriate within the context of that particular placement. This will of course vary and even the same type of placement may need the student to reconsider their appearance a little. This is not the time in your career to be making a fashion statement. It can be a distraction for both the client group and the team members.
- *The student is interested.* Not all placements will be enjoyed by all students. You may actively dislike the area of nursing in which you are temporarily placed. Your role here is to extract the maximum learning opportunities while taking into account the needs of the patients/clients and the established care team. This is regardless of whether you like it or not. It is impressive if you can be proactive about this rather than passive.

Discussion point

When and how could you do this and still maintain some personal sense of continuity and moving forward within the placement? How can you obtain the maximum learning opportunities?

- *The student is approachable and approaching.* It is not up to the mentor or assessor to motivate you through a placement. You do this. You do it regardless of your personal level of motivation at that time. You attempt to create a personal ambience of approachability rather than seeming aloof.
- *The student has a basic appreciation, before they start, of what the placement's goals/philosophies/aims are in respect of their client group.* This will be

addressed in the pre-placement school setting but, if for any reason it isn't, then approach the placement staff and sort this out yourself. It demonstrates that you are trying to respect what it is that the placement staff are trying to achieve.

- *The student manages their personal difficulties.* If you have personal difficulties sometime during the course – and many students do (Wright and Giddey 1993) – then your responsibility is to try to manage this rather than cope (see below).

Expectations of the student

All students going to any placement will have the following expectations of the people who work within that setting ... but sometimes it doesn't work out like that.

- *The staff will be welcoming.* A named individual to contact, who is expecting you, should be sorted out. This helps to diffuse, a little, the usual first-day anxiety that most students experience. (Very occasionally this doesn't happen for a range of reasons, and this is very difficult for all parties involved.) This individual should be able to give you an induction pack, if appropriate, and spend some time on an induction programme. It doesn't have to take very long and the needs of most students are in many ways generic. Being introduced to a small number of the key members of the team is also helpful for all. Also, some idea of how the first week will look is useful and reassuring.
- *The staff will tell you what to expect of them.* This is both in terms of the shape of the week for you and what you are likely to experience in terms of exposure to, and experience with, clients. For example, it is useful to be aware of regularly occurring events such as case meetings, consultant's rounds and so on. It is also useful to be aware of any particularly challenging or demanding clients so that you can prepare, or be prepared, for when you meet them. The staff will warn you of any potential pitfalls, based on the experiences of previous students.
- *The staff will tell you what they expect of you.* This could cover areas such as working hours and any unusual needs on your part for flexibility, depending on the needs of the clients served by that placement team. This will often be reciprocated by a degree of flexibility on the part of the placement staff, if and when you need some extra study time to finish an assignment or collect your poorly child from the nursery. You may also be given some indication of the level of autonomy you are likely to have while on this placement. That is, some assessors will be happy to supervise you at a distance. For example, is there a possibility that you may be given a small supervised caseload of your own, or will the actual face-to-face contact with clients be limited because of the nature of the client group, or some other factor?
- *The staff will have some empathy with the role of the student.* Some staff you work with on placement may be recently qualified. Others may have been working in that speciality for many years. Whatever a carer's length of service, it is very helpful to students if members of the placement team attempt to show some empathy with the student and the different pressures that they are under (this must, of course, be reciprocated). In many ways the expectations of today's students are very different from those of only a few years ago, but even

so the attempt to understand is still very helpful. Surprisingly, some staff who have recently qualified seem to very quickly forget what the student experience is like, whereas some more experienced team members are able to tune into the needs of the student very empathically.

- *The staff will try to accommodate your needs as an individual.* These may be straightforward, in terms of completing pre-set objectives. Some assessors may need to be a little creative about this if opportunities to achieve are not readily available. Some students will really struggle with the academic side of the course, in areas such as connecting theory to practice. Assistance from an experienced assessor who uses 'evidence' to base their practice on is always very helpful with this. Often students will be not only struggling to meet the demands of the course, they will also be trying to meet the demands of their life outside the course.

Given that most contemporary professional carers are also battling to manage large caseloads, understaffed clinical areas and their own personal and academic struggles, supporting the poorly coping student is another pressure that some find almost impossible to manage successfully day in, day out. It is necessary for you to find a strategy to manage your own difficulties without pushing them on to placement care team members.

Some ways of managing this could be to discuss the situation with your:

- Assessor
- Personal tutor
- University counsellor
- GP
- Parent
- Partner
- Friend.

You may wish, of course, to do it the other way around and start with your friend. Some situations will need a problem-solving approach, others will be helped by just talking about it. Some will need a bit of both. Some situations may not have an obvious resolution but may be eased a little by talking about it. Others may need you to have time away from the course with the option of returning. Whatever the difficulty, if it is impacting on your performance as a student, and therefore directly or indirectly on client care, then you must start to address it. A danger if you don't, is that your performance may be judged inaccurately by the people you are working with at that time. In the job of mental health caring you tend to meet the same people many times but in different settings. The people who judge you as a student will carry that judgement until they meet you again. This can colour the relationships you have with other professionals and can work in your favour, or work against you, when you are trying to integrate yourself into a range of different care teams, over the life of your career.

Some commonly experienced student anxieties

Fear of violence

This is a fear of some students who are about to go on to mental health place-ments (see also section 1.19). Many feel uncomfortable or embarrassed to mention it. Some are quite open about it. It is important that students are given reassurance that is honest and direct, and based on fact rather than anecdote or fantasy. Students are probably right to have some reservations. Publicly available evidence suggests that violence is increasing in our wider society and that this is reflected in attacks on health workers (Nhiwatiwa 2003, Thomas *et al.* 1997, Beer *et al.* 2001). The stigma of mental illness may also cause people to draw their own conclusions about increasing violence from the mentally ill.

The reality is that attacks, of course, do happen in mental health clinical areas (Whittington 1992, Baxter 1992) but carers in these areas are probably safer than they have ever been because of the widespread use of personal alarms (Beer *et al.* 2001), increased use of evidence-based risk assessment tools and greater realism when constructing personal safety policies. The influence of factors like these cannot be denied.

It cannot be over-emphasised, however, that the greatest safety device in any clinical area is a vigilant carer. This applies to all levels of staff regardless of grade. It is likely that the most poorly paid, lowest clinically graded health-care workers and students are the ones that are most likely to be near the start of the build-up to a violent incident, as they are the ones that spend the most time with patients (Department of Health 2002a). The great majority of violent incidents in mental health clinical areas do not happen in an instant (Thomas *et al.* 1997, McCarty 1992, Murdach 1993, McSee 1985). Usually there is a build-up to the flash-point. The alert carer will spot the non-verbal cues that indicate this and, if personal intervention is not the most effective response, then getting assistance is the next best strategy.

An essential issue in situations like this is to make your own personal safety the top priority. Do not assume that your relationship with a patient/client will save you, or get you out of trouble. A very small number of mental health carers have even been murdered by the client with whom they thought they had a working relationship (Annis and Baker 1986). *Listen to your intuition, gut feeling, sixth sense, or whatever you like to call it. Respond to that first and intellectualise your reaction later on, when you are in safer conditions.*

Worrying about what you have heard on the grapevine
All institutional work settings have a grapevine system of communication. Sometimes these systems are very accurate. What you hear informally often comes about formally, later on. This happens as the result of people 'in the know' leaking information deliberately or otherwise. You may ask students who have previously been on a placement what it is like. You may ask them what your mentor is like. You may ask them what the patients are like. You will almost always get an opinion. Be clear that this opinion is the result of a person's subjective experience and that this may be different from your own subjective experience. It may be a little different or it may be vastly different. When asked the same questions in the future you may find yourself giving entirely different responses.

You will not stop worrying about what you hear on the grapevine regarding colleagues, policies, clinical areas and so on. After all it may be true. Be aware that it also may not be true. Try to suspend your own judgement until you have experienced things for yourself. Do not even trust first impressions totally, as you may change your mind completely (Burnard 1992). Draw your own conclusions based on as much objective observation as you can. That is, after all, what effective mental health carers do.

Returning to a placement you didn't enjoy first time around

This is often accompanied by a sinking heart and the renewing of negative thoughts and feelings of defeat, resignation ('I'll just have to get through it'). You could view it in a very different way, as a challenge to generate more learning. You could look at the way you manage yourself in difficult situations. You could work on finding the positive aspects to working with clients with whom you find it difficult to empathise. You could reflect on how to work more effectively with colleagues who seem preoccupied and distant. Bear in mind that these strategies could be applied to a placement that may be unchanged since the last time you worked there. The reality is that, over a very short time, in today's mental-health-care settings, staff change, clients change, even environments change. Add to this that you will have changed also. You may find that your second experience is markedly different. The approach used here, to look again at the situation, is an exact replica of the approach used when you work cognitively with your clients, known as 're-framing' (Egan 2002, Altschuler 1997).

Juggling achievement of clinical objectives with assignment work

It is often the experience of students that they see the production of written assignments as a tedious 'hoop' that needs to be jumped through. The assignments are sometimes left until the last minute because of the difficulties involved in achieving clinical objectives on placement, living a life outside the care setting, and avoiding the discomfort necessary in the preparation of the assignment.

As above, a cognitive approach can be constructively used to review this situation. Given that all nurses are guided by their Code of Conduct (NMC) to work using evidence-based practice, the process of searching through a range of resources to obtain recent research and literature findings is a helpful discipline to develop. The way that the assignments should be written, in coherent, objective English, is also a good training for the discipline of writing coherent objective observations about your clients in their care plans. The deadlines you are given, by which time a piece of work must be handed in, is a good training for the discipline of meeting deadlines in the clinical world – e.g. the giving of a patient's once-monthly injection, the production of a report for a care meeting, the completion of a staffing rota to cover a holiday period, the completion of your CV for your next promotion by the advertised closing date. The production of these assignments is a rehearsal for the carrying out of your role as a qualified nurse. The discipline required is similar.

Juggling achievement of clinical objectives, completion of assignments to the right level and domestic/personal problems

With few exceptions, this is a familiar scenario to mental health students. Some students seem to go through this combination of difficulties in patches, while others seem to be dogged by problems throughout their course.

For some the course itself brings its own difficulties. The selfishness and self-centredness needed to be a successful student can cause or exacerbate domestic tensions that perhaps were not apparent before, or could be managed or ignored prior to the start of the course. The good luck of being in a group of students in school who are motivated, interested and engaged with the material can expedite and encourage learning. The bad luck of being in a disparate collection of individuals with their own agendas can have the opposite effect. Some teaching staff will see this and try to address it. Others will not see it, or will choose to ignore it.

The skill of completing assignments to the appropriate academic standard, together with searching for tutorial staff to help with tutorials, is difficult. The strain of being around patients and clients who are often challenging in different ways, combined with trying to be professional and competent in yet another new group of professionals, can seem relentless. Altogether, this can mean that the course is uniquely tiring and stressful.

Over the stretch of a 3-year course, life will throw up challenges for every student that may or may not be directly connected to the course. Child care difficulties, pregnancy, illness, financial problems worsened by trying to live on a bursary, accommodation, relationship problems, travelling, working on shifts, road accidents, bereavements – the list goes on.

Your training institution will no doubt offer a support service in some form. This could be a student support or counselling service. There may be short-term financial support available. Overseas students may find that they have access to specialists who can help and advise with work permits and visas. Your personal tutor may be able to help directly or guide you to someone who will be able to do so. Some are very experienced at helping students through these difficult patches. Your mentor may be able to offer support in a different way from your school contact, especially if the nature of your problem is more clinically orientated.

All students are entitled to belong to a union. This may be your local branch of the Student's Union or one of the nursing or care worker unions (see Appendix B). A local representative from one of these bodies may be able to help you. Your own group of students, or even students ahead of you on the course, may be a strong source of support for you.

Besides all this, there are organisations such as Relate, Parentline, the Samaritans, NHS Direct, Citizens Advice, and so on (see Appendix B), depending on the nature of your difficulty. Your GP may also be able to help if the root of your difficulty is a physical or mental illness that needs to be addressed.

The personal experience of the author suggests that, when these problems become apparent, the most effective course of action is to address them at an early stage, before things get out of hand and become often more difficult, painful, or embarrassing to address. Take a deep breath and ring up or (e-mail) your personal tutor, college counsellor, assessor, GP or whoever it is who seems to be the most appropriate.

Going to a placement you *know* you are not going to like
You could decide to maintain this way of thinking or you could decide to reserve judgement. The reasons for this, and ways of doing it, are elaborated on above. A negative approach to any placement may result in a self-fulfilling prophecy (Adler and Towne 1999). In other words, what you expect is more likely to happen. You have nothing to lose by approaching your placement determined to get

something positive out of it for yourself. Your personal tutor or mentor may be able to help with this 're-framing'. Also, many students (in my experience) seem to experience a heightened level of learning in challenging, difficult or 'uncomfortable' placements.

Wondering if you will be able to perform at the 'right level'

The right level can be the level of a first year student, a second year student, a staff nurse or just the students who were your predecessors. The gauging of the right level will be done by many different people.

- *The nursing care team*. They may help to support the view of your assessor or mentor or they may disagree with it. It is essential to listen to their feedback, even if sometimes it is uncomfortable. What you are hearing may represent how you are seen by other groups of professionals. This matters because as long as you are a professional mental health carer, you will *never* be working in isolation. You will need to have the ability to be a team worker.
- *Other professionals*. This is similar to the views above. It is essential that the effective nurse has the ability to work in a mixed professional group with as little tension as possible while at the same time being professionally assertive (see section 3.4). The care a client receives will be affected by the co-ordinated approach and consistency of the team that is helping them. Tensions within care teams are almost invariably transmitted to the focus of their care – the client. The team of professionals you work with on each placement will be making informal and formal judgements about you, regardless of their role, grade or speciality.
- *Your assessor or mentor*. Using their experience and professional judgement, they will compare your performance to the objectives book you will have with you. They will consult with other professionals. The comments you receive will be a consensus view of several team members. The relationship you have with your assessor can help to make your experience positive and enhance the quality of your learning. It will pay you to invest in this relationship, even though it is temporary. Work as much as possible with them. Make allowances when they are too busy or preoccupied to make you the centre of attention. Try to be creative and helpful. Use your initiative. Always try to stretch your abilities while staying within your personal and clinical limitations. An effective mentor will help you define just what these are.
- *The clients*. It is unlikely that clients will be asked to assess your ability as a student, although some clients are on interview panels to recruit new mental health carers, so it is not impossible. They will, however, be gauging your effectiveness, taking into consideration that you are a student and therefore do not have the authority of a staff nurse. You will become aware that, as you spend more time in the placement, more and more clients seek you out for help, advice, assistance with practical things or just a chat. The more this happens the more you are being accepted as an effective carer. It is prudent, however, not to try to artificially accelerate this process. Pace yourself. If you are doing it right, the clients will seek you out.
- *Their friends and relatives*. You will quickly realise that the client's relatives and significant others are an informal part of the care team, for better or

worse. Some relatives are supportive and loving. Others are sabotaging and destructive. Whatever their relationship with, and impact on, the client, their needs also have to be taken into account within any care strategy. Given that, it is also important that you take account of the judgements this group of people will be making about you.

- *You.* Your objective measure of how you are doing is the book listing your aims/goals that you take to your placement, and the comments on it from your assessor. Your subjective measures are the things people say to you as you go about your work, and the voice in your head that validates your performance or criticises it. All these need to be listened to.

Objectively the only one of the above list that matters to you as a student is your professional assessor. Subjectively they all matter, and the ones that matter most of all are the clients.

Thinking 'The course is nearly ended – and I don't know anything'
You do. If you are nearly at the end of the course, the assessment system will almost certainly have ensured that you are somewhere near the appropriate level of a starting-grade nurse. Also it may surprise you that you have learned some things by osmosis. When you start as a qualified nurse there is a vast amount of information to be accessed, processed and stored. In the first few weeks, you will be introduced every day to new material and new uncertainties. It will feel different to you because now you carry the full responsibility that your registration gives you. The task you have is to make sure you know what is essential and not to worry so much about the issues that can wait until some other time.

Your new colleagues can help you with this. They have all been through the same process. The skills of communicating effectively with all people who you encounter professionally have never been more important as you try to establish yourself in your new professional team.

1 THE RUDIMENTS

The skills, techniques and ideas in this chapter can be the basis of every professional intervention you make. They can be relied upon to help you in any intervention with patients/clients in any setting. The level is appropriate for the first year student to attempt, under supervision.

1.1 JUST LISTENING

Most books on interpersonal skills are likely to contain a section on 'listening skills' and in that sense this book is no different. There is value, however, in stressing to the newcomer to mental health nursing (and any other kind of carer) not to underestimate the helping potential of just listening, or that is how it will probably look to the person who is talking. As the sections below will make clear, there is much more to it than that. The art of listening is just like any other art. When you see it carried out by an expert it looks easy, almost as if nothing is happening.

This is a theme that recurs throughout this book. For example the point is made later on that the 'expert' mental health nurse can often carry out an assessment interview making it look as if an everyday conversation is taking place. There is great benefit in this to the patient/client. They are more likely to be as relaxed as possible in what is often a difficult and uneasy situation: 'Service users report that the process of admission can itself be a distressing and demeaning experience' (Department of Health 2002a, p. 12). If they feel relatively relaxed, and therefore relatively safe and in control, they are more able to talk in an open way to the assessing mental health carer, if they choose to do so.

So what is just listening? The word 'just' implies lack of importance but nothing could be further from the truth. Think of the last time someone really listened to you when you were troubled by something. It is likely that this happens quite rarely. If your listener was really listening, and not constantly pushing in with bits of their own conversation, it is possible that you felt a little better at the end of the conversation than at the beginning. So what did this listening person contribute to the conversation? What were the characteristics that seemed to be most helpful?

Discussion point

Think of a person who you have found to be helpful to you in terms of their ability to listen. What are they like? What can you learn from them?

The helpful person

It is probable that the person was something like this:

- They were quiet for most of the conversation. The balance of the talking was heavily weighted towards you
- They were encouraging. They nodded as if they understood and followed what you were saying. They might have smiled occasionally, but only if this helped you
- They looked at you as if they were interested, without staring
- They were sitting or standing in a similar way to you and at a comfortable distance away from you, not too near or too far away
- They looked reasonably relaxed, depending on what it was that you were talking about
- They occasionally asked you to go over something again briefly to make sure that they really understood
- They might sometimes briefly repeat back to you a summary of what you had just said to make sure that they understood you
- They might sometimes say things to you that caused you to think 'This person really does understand me'
- You felt that whatever you said you would not be judged. Therefore you could say anything. This felt very liberating
- You felt that this person respected you regardless of the differences between you.

As the listener you will often know when you have demonstrated most of the above characteristics. The other person will say something like: 'Thanks for listening ... that feels better'. Or they may say nothing but will look a little less tense, a little more relaxed.

1.2 THE IMPORTANCE OF THOUGHTFUL COMMUNICATION

'Thoughtful' is used here to indicate that the nurse is thinking about what they are doing all the time they are with the patient, even if nothing much seems to be happening. The thoughtfulness may not be immediately apparent to the patient. This is the area of care in which the mental health nurse can make a difference to patients/clients on a daily basis, given the desire, motivation and energy.

It doesn't matter if you are a student nurse or a staff nurse of many years' experience. Paradoxically, the literature consistently records that the latter has much less time to do this (Whittington and McLaughlin 2000). The time you spend listening to, and talking with, the people in your care can matter and make a difference to them. Doing this can change their experience of being ill, usually for the better (this is not guaranteed, however).

It is important to note here that sometimes the *attempt* can be almost as valuable to the patient as the content of your intervention. They may experience some of the following, if you at least try to communicate thoughtfully:

- *Having thoughts or feelings validated.* This means that the person is likely to feel that in some way their thoughts or feelings were/are appropriate and acceptable, given their personal and unique set of circumstances. This is also supportive and may provide some comfort. For example:

  Sonia. I really regret leaving the way I did. I hurt so many people.
  Nurse. You probably did what seemed to be best at the time. People can be surprisingly resilient sometimes.

- *Having the sense that someone has an inkling of what they are going through*. This can be the start of empathy. Empathy is discussed later on (section 2.11) but for now it can be understood as the ability of the nurse to communicate to the patient the sense that they have some idea of what the patient is experiencing or has experienced For example:

> Sonia. Yes, but it still troubles me even after all this time.
> Nurse. You sound worn down with it all.
> Sonia. That's spot on, I am.

- *Having a friend*. 'It is important to be clear that, although we are sometimes friendly professionals, we are not professional friends' (Jackson 1998, see also McGovern and Whitcher 1994). It is important that whenever possible we are friendly and approachable, but professional. This is rather than pretending to be friendly because we feel that it is necessary as part of our job. For example:

> Sonia. I feel so alone at the moment, like I've lost everything.
> Nurse. You know we're here for you, whenever you need to talk? Any of the team will be happy to spend some time with you.

- *Being noticed*. For example:

> Sonia. It seems like people have forgotten I exist. No one visits any more.
> Nurse. You seem to be withdrawing from everyone, though. How about ringing your sister – she was asking about you, wasn't she?

- *Having someone on their side*. Again, this involves being supportive. For example:

> Sonia. Yes but she's not really bothered. She does it out of duty.
> Nurse. You could give it a try; you might be surprised. You are her only sister, after all.

- *Not feeling so alone*. People who suffer from all forms of mental illness can feel this way (Barker *et al.* 2000). For example:

> Sonia. I spend hours on my own just trying to work out what went wrong. My brain is spinning.
> Nurse. Let's talk it through for a while? It might help you untangle things.

- *Having someone to listen to unacceptable thoughts – and be accepting*. Acceptance is a very important component of the effective nurse–patient relationship. The patient must feel accepted, not judged, by the nurse, otherwise they are less likely to feel that they can talk about what is really happening for them. For example:

> Sonia. Sometimes I wish I could go to sleep and not wake up again. At least I'd get away from this mess.
> Nurse. I suppose that is an answer, but what would it be like for the people you leave behind?

Thoughtful communication can help patients (sometimes) to express these things. If this happens, the nurse has been effective both in a short-term and a longer-term way. In the short term the person may feel relief, or at least some change in emotional or feeling state. Even if their state is worsened, and sometimes this can happen, the issues are nearer the surface and can be accessed by the nurse. This could be a useful opportunity to work on material that is the real truth for some patients.

This is a point at which nurses, whether student or newly qualified, needs to be aware of their limitations. When this situation arises, it is not a foregone conclusion that the 'beginner' nurse has to quickly back out. As long as the nurse acknowledges to the patient that they may be getting near to the edge of their experience, why not try it? For example:

> **Nurse.** I've not been in this situation before, but if it's OK with you, we could keep talking about your situation. I'll need to speak to my supervisor afterwards, though, to check I've done the right thing.

Here the nurse is being open about their limitations while at the same time asking for consent from the patient to carry on, or not. In addition, the nurse is able to give the patient some reassurance that they have access to someone else who may be able to help. These opportunities can be really valuable in terms of developing the depth of experience.

Talking to a mentor can be very helpful at points like this. It is very helpful to try and arrange regular sessions where clinical work with patients and its professional and personal impact can be discussed. These sessions may be known as 'supervision' and are a characteristic of well-planned mental health teams (Veeramah 2002). Discussing the dialogue, in supervision, can help clarify and validate early experiences, which are often very memorable and form a constructive template of experience that can be used over and over again. For example:

> **Student nurse.** It really upset me when Sonia was talking about her family. It reminded me so much of that other patient who was here a few months ago.
> **Mentor.** Yes, and remember how you came to terms with what happened to him?

In the longer term, the basis of a relationship is being put down, layer by layer. This can be used in the future to help the patient.

The future, by the way, can be later that day, next month or in several years time. The job of mental health nursing often seems to involve meeting the same people over and over again. We all get older and the settings change, but the relationships you start now can last for a very long time. At its very best, the relationship is like a bank account that is earning compound interest. Over time it can become more valuable in terms of its potential help.

An issue that can separate the more experienced thoughtful communicator from the less experienced is the degree of intention (Heron 2001; see also section 2.2) The more experienced thoughtful carer has an idea of how to help the patient at any particular time, both at that moment and over a longer period. This is not to suggest that the nurse is leading the direction of the conversation. Sometimes, being directive can be helpful, but only as a result of really listening to the patient in as nearly empathic a manner as possible (Rogers 1951, Egan 2002, Nelson Jones 2002). Even if that directiveness turns out to be not right for the patient, it could be suggested that this is still progress in terms of processing through a range of ideas or options (Egan 2002) to discount the inappropriate.

1.3 THE DIFFERENCES BETWEEN THOUGHTFUL AND THOUGHTLESS COMMUNICATION

The main difference here is again, the idea of 'intention' (Heron 2001). Experienced nurses are more likely to achieve their intention more often than less experienced ones. However, there is no guarantee of this. It is worth bearing in mind that sometimes even an apparently disastrous interaction or intervention can be used to help the patient if it is managed constructively and imaginatively. Often student nurses express their anxiety about 'saying the wrong thing' to patients (see also section 1.14). Look at the following example:

> **Student nurse.** Hi, Edith – is your husband visiting tonight?
> **Edith.** There's no way I want that bastard anywhere near me. He's the reason I'm in this nuthouse.
> **Student nurse.** Oh sorry – I didn't realise.

This looks as if the attempt to make light conversation with Edith has gone wrong. However the skilled nurse has been presented here with an opportunity to work with what might be 'fresh' emotional material. This is congruent with some of the literature on crisis intervention, which describes a crisis as an opportunity (Gibson 1991, Johnstone 2000). The original intention was to find out basic information and also develop a rapport, or in other words an increase in the easiness of the communication The actual response seems to contain both information and a sense of catharsis (the expression of emotions or feelings). Either of these are valuable for the nurse to work with, in terms of helping Edith to move forward. The two combined possibly have greater therapeutic potential in terms of helping the nurse see how Edith feels.

See how the nature of this interaction can be changed, using the same starting point:

> **Nurse.** Hi, Edith – is your husband visiting tonight?
> **Edith.** There's no way I want that bastard anywhere near me. He's the reason I'm in this nuthouse.
> **Nurse.** Oh, sorry, I didn't realise that was the situation. What happened?
> **Edith.** He left me for a woman at his work. I couldn't cope. He didn't care.
> **Nurse.** What do you mean, he didn't care?
> **Edith.** He never came to see me at the hospital. He didn't even phone.
> **Nurse.** You say he didn't care. Could there be any other reasons that he didn't phone?

The nurse is gently and tentatively taking Edith into territory that otherwise might not have been explored. She is making the most of an opportunity that otherwise would perhaps be seen as a mistake.

1.4 BEING APPROACHABLE

A primary ingredient of thoughtful interventions is that the nurse needs to be approachable by the patient.

Some characteristics of this are:

- Being friendly (sometimes this is difficult, but you try)
- Acknowledging people (this is never difficult)
- Looking relaxed (can be difficult sometimes).

These three components are likely to maximise, but not guarantee, the chances that people may choose to talk to you. This is important when the literature suggests that patients' perceptions are that nurses are too busy to talk. Objectively, research has consistently demonstrated that mental health nurses don't spend much time talking to patients (Whittington and McLaughlin 2000).

As a beginner it is important that you spend some time discussing and reflecting with your assessors, colleagues, teachers, fellow students, and even some of the patients/clients (if it is appropriate), what makes you approachable. With patients this could be a good way to learn this skill anyway. If you are approachable, then at least the patient has the choice to start to engage with you or not, rather than no choice at all. Also, the time when you are a student is the best time to exploit this opportunity, as once you become a qualified nurse your relationship with patients/clients will be different.

1.5 WHY YOUR SELF-AWARENESS MATTERS TO OTHERS

As with listening skills, most books on interpersonal skills will address self-awareness. How do we become more self-aware and why should we bother anyway? The literature around this area suggests that first impressions are highly significant to us in general social situations (Burnard 1992, p. 17). Think how much more significant this becomes when placed in mental health settings?

Discussion point

What consequences could first impressions have for a patient/client when meeting a nurse for the first time. How could this be different for a nurse meeting a patient/client for the first time?

There are many aspects to this:

- How do you look?
- What do you say?
- How do you behave?
- How do you seem (subjectively) to the other person?
- What does the whole situation feel like (subjectively) to you?
- Are you still 'open' afterwards?
- What is your reputation?

How do you look?

Many learners are referred to Egan's (2002) acronym **SOLER**:

Sitting with an
Open posture
Leaning forward, using appropriate
Eye contact and being
Relaxed.

You don't need to have worked in mental health care for very long to realise that this model should not be taken too literally. Probably, Egan's intention was to use this as a starting point only. The usefulness of this acronym is to remind us that we should be aware of our presentation to the patient/client. Ask yourself: 'What is this person seeing when they look at me?' Are they seeing someone who looks approachable, interested, and willing to engage? On the other hand, are they looking at someone who is preoccupied, distracted, agitated or not really interested? Is the patient likely to be distracted, repelled or attracted by your clothing (Arnold and Boggs 2003), hairstyle, accessories and general demeanour? At what point does this not matter, because the attention is focused on what you are saying and doing, rather than how you look? Or does it always matter?

As always these are complex issues and, at the time of writing some clinical areas have reverted to wearing uniform instead of everyday clothing. How the effects of this can be meaningfully measured is not clear. The issue is that it does matter how you look, as this is the first piece of communication you send to every new patient/client that you meet. (This does not include writing to, or phoning, patients/clients and others. These are of course essential and skilled pieces of communication – see also sections 1.18 and 2.21.)

What do you say?

An assumption is made that you appear to be approachable (section 1.4) and that you are aware of the need to create a rapport (section 1.7), which includes telling the patient/client who you are and what you are doing. The next stage can be something like this.

> **Nurse.** How's it going?/How did you get on at the weekend?/How are you settling in?/When are you due to see Dr Campbell again?

You will note that all the above interventions use open questions (section 2.8). These are questions that use words such as when/where/why/how/what? These words provide an invitation to the other person. The invitation may not be accepted straight away, but part of your role is to keep providing the opportunities. Whatever the response is to each invitation, you have more assessment data that you can use to help the patient.

How do you behave?

You must behave in a welcoming way. In a way that does not dis-empower, intimidate, or belittle. In an accepting way. In a way that you can sustain. In a way that is consistent. In a way that is congruent – in other words, how you *seem* is how you *are*.

How do you seem?

This looks at the objective and subjective experience of the patient/client. All of us probably experience what psychotherapists would describe as 'transferences' (Varcarolis 1998). We need to consider the transferences of the patient/client. Who do we remind them of at a conscious or subconscious level? They see us, they hear us, they probably feel something about us. This can be liking, feeling comfortable with, trusting or the opposite of all these. To a great extent we cannot control how people feel about us. In the professional mental health setting we can have some influence over this, bearing in mind, and reminding ourselves, that this is entirely for the benefit of our patient.

What does the whole situation feel like?

You will often have some sense of: 'This is going well/this feels uncomfortable/I feel awkward/I feel confident....' it is interesting to reflect on the reasons for these thoughts and feelings afterwards, either on your own or preferably in a supervision session with your mentor. You can sometimes learn much about yourself, the patient/client and the nature of your relationships with them.

Are you still 'open' afterwards?

In other words, after your first meeting with the patient/client, whether it is at the drugs trolley, during their admission to your ward or on their front doorstep at their initial assessment, do they still feel OK to 'approach' you, in every sense? Do they feel OK to phone you on the ward if they are 'on leave' (if this is one of the conditions of your relationship)? Do they feel OK to approach you in the ward office, which is your own territory, to catch you in between phone calls to social workers, psychiatrists and solicitors? Do they feel OK to phone your base if you are working in a community setting?

What is your reputation?

Where does it come from? How can you influence it? Do you want to? You will become aware very quickly that some nurses/carers are seen as approachable and good listeners. Others are seen as standoffish and unapproachable. It is important early in your career to work out which of these you want to be and why. You can take steps to convert from one to the other at any stage in your career as a mental health nurse.

1.6 Intuition

Gut feeling, sixth sense or whatever you wish to call it is both rudimentary and sophisticated. As far as the beginner nurse is concerned, it is important to listen to your intuition and react to it – i.e. to consider doing what it tells you. You may find out that your intuition is sometimes wrong, but it is unlikely to harm you to listen and sometimes respond to what it tells you. It can, however, be very dangerous to ignore your intuition and attempt to intellectualise its message by dismissing it as nonsense. For example; you are sitting in the day room having a conversation with Patrick, a patient with whom you've developed a good rapport. The dialogue feels easy, open and warm. During a natural break in the conversation you glance around you and notice that a newly admitted male patient is steadily staring at you, in what feels to you like a threatening manner.

   You have some options here:

1 Continue your easy conversation
2 Engage the new patient in conversation
3 Leave the area for a while.

Intellectually, you might choose options 1 or 2, but *intuitively* you might choose option 3.

Intellectually you might be thinking:

- *Option 1.* It's easy and safe to talk to Patrick. He always appreciates the time I spend with him. It's my job anyway.
- *Option 2.* I'll talk to the new chap. He makes me feel uneasy, so I'll confront my fear. It'll be all right.

Your intuition may be saying to you:

- *Option 3.* I don't like the look of this chap at all. I'm not sure what he's going to do. He frightens me a bit. I'm leaving the area.

Option 1 would probably be taken by nurses who feel a little uncertain about their ability to create a rapport with the new patient and choose the security of the 'known'.

Option 2 would probably be taken by more experienced nurses who feel safe in their environment and confident that they know how to create a rapport with threatening or unknown patients. They would also know they could get help quickly by using a personal alarm. Personal alarms are now issued to carers in many mental health areas as a matter of course. Occasionally, mental health carers are attacked and injured, sometimes badly. Very occasionally they are killed. The use of alarms is one reaction to these relatively rare incidents.

Option 3 would be taken by nurses who are following their instinct. Out of the three this is possibly the best beginner's choice, for the following reasons.

To continue talking with Patrick is to ignore what might be a situation about to fly out of control. To directly engage the new patient when he is unknown to you and looking (apparently) threateningly towards you takes a high level of skill and confidence. The best course of action for the beginner is to leave the area quickly and quietly. The assistance of an experienced member of staff, who should be better placed to know the most appropriate intervention with an unknown and apparently threatening patient, can be sought.

This may seem unsatisfactory to more experienced readers. There are some indications that nurses do trust their intuition, but there can be difficulties with this: 'Intuition was seen by many … to play an important part in assessing the risk of violence. The problem here is that intuition varies from person to person' (Doyle 1996, p. 22). Also, Arnold and Boggs (2003, p. 247) suggest that: 'Nurses need to listen to their intuitive feelings, but it is also important to validate this intuitive knowledge with the client to fully understand the meaning of the behaviour (of the client)'. We sometimes never know what would have been the best course of action. But sometimes we find out too late what wasn't. Many violent incidents in institutional mental health settings can be 'nipped in the bud' by effective nursing interventions before they get out of hand.

1.7 STARTING A RAPPORT

Sometimes this is very easy; sometimes it is excruciatingly difficult. This can depend on a combination of many things:

- The setting
- The conditions of the first meeting

- The resistance of the patient – this can be linked to their mental health difficulty, their natural (premorbid) personality, or both
- Your familiarity with the territory
- The pressure you are under to create the rapport.

Let us look at the worst possible scenario first.

Institutional setting

You are a first-year student, who has just met your assessor/mentor on the first day of your first psychiatric placement. He seems rather distracted and says: 'Nice to meet you. I'm a bit tied up at the moment … go and talk to the patients. I'll catch up with you in a bit.'

Where do you start? How do you do it? What do you say? Why are you doing it anyway?

It could be quite in order at this point to make a cup of tea or coffee for yourself, pick up a magazine/paper and then go to see where some of the patients are. This is most likely to be a day room or 'smoking area'. As you become a little more experienced you will quickly realise that this is one of the best places to carry out unobtrusive observation. As you approach them and before you get too near (even patients on their own) say something like: 'Hi/good morning/good afternoon/hello I'm Martin/Lynne. I'm a student nurse here for the next few weeks. OK if I join you for a bit?'

It is important to say *who you are*, *what your role is* in the care team and *how long you are likely to be around*. Look at it from the patients' point of view. They are likely to feel differently about you if you are:

- Male or female
- Younger, the same age, or older than them
- Here for one day or three months
- A student nurse, a qualified nurse, a social worker, a health care assistant, a volunteer.

Wearing the institution's name badge, if appropriate, is also useful to help patients locate you in the organisational structure. The importance of this for the patient is that your position carries with it a degree of responsibility and authority. Knowledge about this will help some patients select you (or not) to help them. For example, the more experienced patients will know that it is a waste of time asking the health care assistant on the ward if they can go home for the weekend, unless that is the way they usually access the staff who are 'too busy'.

In many instances, patients will be:

- Curious as to who you are, and why you are there
- Ambivalent
- Pleased to see you and to have some different company – patients are often very bored (Polemeni *et al.* 1992)
- Non-reactive (apparently).

What you could do then is to sit down somewhere nearby, but not too close, and start to read the paper and drink your tea. This is how it looks anyway. Of course, what is happening is much more sophisticated and subtle, and again intention-driven.

The cup of tea and the paper are acting as comfort barriers both for you, and the new people you are about to meet. It is something for you to hold and something for you to do, to get you through the awkward social silences that are a feature of the beginning of many institutional nurse–patient relationships. It is probably good that you feel awkward. Maybe it would be a little inappropriate to feel completely confident and in control at this stage.

The purpose of introducing yourself by your first name and saying you will be here for this shift/day/afternoon is that it is a non-authoritarian way of indicating that you are a paid carer. This is important, as it can be very embarrassing to be mistaken for a patient, for a very specific reason. Disclosures by patients to other patients can sometimes be much more personal than to 'the staff', especially until they get used to you. If you are mistaken for a patient, you may find that boundaries have accidentally/unknowingly been crossed. This can be very embarrassing for both the patient and you.

Once you are established in the proximity of the individual patient, or the group, the actions of reading the paper and drinking tea indicate a democratic/participative 'ordinariness' (see also section 1.9) that is helpful as part of your relationship-building skills repertoire.

After a few minutes the next action is to finish your drink and then perhaps leave the patient group/individual with something like: 'See you later!'

Again this is done deliberately as it leaves an opening for you to return in a few minutes time, later that day, or tomorrow. You then make sure that, after a reasonable time has passed, depending on the setting, you repeat the process again. This time it is likely to be a little easier, and next time a little easier still. The building up of a warm rapport is the first step towards the start (only) of a 'therapeutic relationship' (see also sections 2.10 and 2.11).

Community setting

We will take this as your first visit with a community psychiatric nurse (CPN) to visit a client, with a view to carrying out an initial assessment. The CPN has telephoned ahead to let the client know when you are calling. You call at the house:

> CPN. Hello, Miss Foster, I'm Lynne from the community team, and this is Sharon, a student. We spoke on the phone this morning. Could you spare a few minutes?
>
> Miss Foster. Yes, come in. It's not going to take too long, is it?
>
> CPN. It will take about an hour. Most people find that's enough for a first meeting and that's about as much information as I can handle anyway. Just say if it's getting too much and we'll stop. How does that sound to you?

The intention here is to give the first meeting some limits or parameters. There has been a demonstration of a level of experience and expertise that is realistic and not overblown. There has been a small self-disclosure. The client is empowered (or at least the attempt has been made). The feelings of the client are monitored. Overall this is an effective interaction. It is short, focused, client centred and intention-driven.

The next bit is the start of the development of the rapport building. Some options are as follows:

> 'It's cold out, isn't it?'
> 'Your garden's looking good.'
> 'Where can I sit?'
> 'How have things been for you lately?'
> 'Your GP wrote to the team and said … (*quotes parts of the referral letter*). What do you think of that?'
> 'Could you tell me how we could start to help you?'
> 'Could you talk me through what's been happening?'

You will notice that some of the early suggestions above are apparently more to do with rapport, and the later ones are more about getting on with the job. This is probably a reflection of the power balance in non-institutional settings, where the client often has a greater sense of control and the carer does not have to tread quite so carefully to ease gently into the process. You have to make a judgement here. Some people will be comfortable for you to get straight on with the 'business'. Others will need a gentler approach. If you are unsure, the safest tactic is to start with a few relatively superficial interactions that are designed to ease into the 'working' part of the interaction:

> 'This is the worst/best/driest/wettest summer/winter that I can remember.'

See how the person reacts to this sort of remark. If they are comfortable at this level then it is OK to tentatively introduce the idea of something more challenging.

> 'I've got a copy of the letter that your GP sent to me. Could we start off by going through it together?'

Often rapport building is a matter of trial and error, but it is an essential stage in the caring process in most clinical settings. Investment at this stage will pay off, as you may find that the patient/client is less resistant to, or more welcoming of, your thoughtful intentions.

Discussion point

How might the environment affect the dynamics between client and professional carer? What are the pros and cons of visiting people in their own homes as opposed to seeing them in a more neutral environment such as the GP surgery?

1.8 BEING NON-INTRUSIVE

In many ways the job of the mental health nurse is to be intrusive. During the assessment process we need to ask questions that sometimes cause discomfort to patients or clients. If our questions are not intrusive then we may not be getting the data from and about the patient/client that will help to facilitate an appropriate treatment plan.

> **Nurse.** So how has your sleep been over the last month, Joan?
> **Joan.** OK – fine, really.

Nurse. You sound a bit unsure.
Joan. Well sometimes I don't sleep much.
Nurse. What do you mean? What's it like when you don't sleep much?
Joan. I wake up at 5 a.m. most mornings.
Nurse. What wakes you?
Joan. My head is spinning. I can't stop thinking about what happened to me.
Nurse. What do you mean?
Joan. Oh, I can't talk about it. Not at the moment anyway.

And this is the moment when, perhaps, the nurse makes the decision to become non-intrusive. The interaction follows the process of obtaining information about Joan's sleeping patterns. Then it diverts into something that is obviously of a more sensitive nature. The instinct of the effective mental health nurse will be to want to find out about what happened to Joan, but at the moment it might feel over-intrusive to Joan. It could be embarrassing, uncomfortable or painful for her to talk about it. Finding out what happened could be vital to formulating a care plan that will work for her. But now is not the time. The skill of the nurse is deciding when *is* the time.

This skill demonstrates clearly a respect for the needs of the patient/client.

1.9 Ordinariness and how it can help

Being ordinary could be an aim, perhaps, of many thoughtful nurses in their interactions with patients. From the patient's point of view, an 'ordinary' conversation is taking place (Barker 2003). This ordinariness presents no threat and may encourage the patient's sense of control. The nurse and patient are a little nearer to an equal relationship, with an equal balance of power (Altschuler 1997). Patients are more likely to say how they really feel in this situation. If this is how it feels to the patient, then the nurse is being effective in terms of trying to *empower* the patient.

Empowering, here, means that patients have the sense of being a little more in control of their destiny (see also section 2.14). If the interaction has this feel, then the patient may be encouraged to be more *independent* and *autonomous* – independent in that they will not willingly become dependent, and autonomous in that they feel they have retained their individuality. They are respected and their dignity has been preserved.

All these terms have a sense of idealism about them. Often in nursing we aim for the ideal but fall short. At least we have tried.

At the other end of the continuum from ordinary interventions are those that seem to contain a solution. These are the territory of the experienced expert and should be avoided by beginners. They are the sentences that seem to contain 'the answer' for the patient. If you find yourself tempted to come up with answers and solutions in this way, it may be useful to consider trying to resist.

Mary. I wish my kids could understand how hard it's been for me. They just don't realise how much of a front I've been putting on all this time.
Nurse. You could always sit down and tell them how you really feel.

This is a 'solution sentence' that contains the acknowledgement of the problem, the action and the 'expert' answer. Alternatively here is an apparently non-expert but possibly more useful response that can be carried on from the one above.

Nurse. But I suppose real life isn't that easy though. What do you reckon?

This is an 'ordinary' add-on that brings the response back down to earth, makes it real and puts the power of discretion back into the hands of the patient. The fuller response also encourages Mary to use her own reasoning to get nearer to her own resolution of her problems.

This is an example of a technique called *Socratic reasoning* (Nelson Jones 1997, Norman and Redfern 1997). Socratic reasoning has its origins in the approach of the Greek philosopher Socrates, who tried to encourage people to work out their own answers to their problems. It is a very useful and widely applicable technique for mental health carers.

Mary. It's going to be really difficult to talk to them. It's something I've never done. I've never talked to them before and told them what's going on.
Nurse (*using a Socratic approach*). How do think you could start things off with them?
Mary. I don't know. This is really difficult
Nurse. What would you be hoping to achieve if things went well?
Mary. I'd like to feel we were a family for once.

Burnard (2003) also suggests that ordinary, or *phatic*, conversation has a useful role in mental health nursing in terms of developing a rapport with the patient or client.

1.10 OBSERVATION IN MENTAL HEALTH SETTINGS

Observation is probably *the* primary skill used by the effective mental health nurse. From the observation comes the intervention. The intervention, as described above, may range from apparently doing nothing tangible to an intervention that is a direct response to what has been observed. As with assessing, the mental health nurse is always observing and trying to make sense of what is happening to patients/clients. What is the significance of their verbal and non-verbal presentation?

The more experienced nurse is probably not aware that they are doing it during much of their working day. It becomes part of the professional persona. It is however probably the most important action that mental health carers carry out. Everything else stems from observation of the people in their care, regardless of the setting.

Observation is part of a more formalised approach when the patient is assessed as being at risk: 'Nurses trained in the appropriate techniques should carry out close observation. It should be recognised that special observation can exacerbate behavioural disturbance and unobtrusive monitoring can sometimes be used effectively' (Beer *et al.* 2001, p. 17). (See also Thompson and Mathias 1994, Newell and Gournay 2000, Ramos, cited in Lego 1996.)

1.11 BEING OPTIMISTIC

Even in the most negative of mental health situations it is part of the nurse's role to be professionally optimistic, constructive and positive. Sometimes this is very difficult, and nurses have to try to change their own personal view in terms of the way they see a patient's or client's situation to something more positive. Many people who need mental health services are feeling defeated in some way. It is important for them that we maintain an assertively supportive and encouraging approach.

Some of the patients/clients we meet seem to be the victims of, or the result of, dysfunctional systems – environments, cultures, groups, families that have a long history of repeating maladaptive patterns of behaviour. We are often reminded that sometimes the people we meet in mental health settings are very damaged by their history. A likelihood is that they return to the same environment that contributed to the damage in the first place. Williamson (2003, p. 26) puts this in an Assertive Outreach setting: 'It is crucial that practitioners maintain a sense of belief and optimism in the potential for recovery'. This philosophy can be transferred into any mental health clinical setting.

Our optimism, then, is often not about people getting better or being cured, it is about them being able to manage a little better, or a little less badly, within their own environment. Egan (2002, p. 261) writes about the hope we need to have as helpers and quotes St Paul: 'Hope that centres around things you can see is not really hope'.

1.12 BEING TENTATIVE

When you work with patients/clients in this way you are feeling your way gently, carefully, sensitively. A tentative approach means that you are less likely to make assumptions or jump to conclusions that may not be true. The more you avoid doing so, the more accurate your assessment of patients and clients is likely to be. This means that the treatment evolving from the assessment is likely to be more effective. Here is an example of a tentative approach in an assessment situation:

Community Psychiatric Nurse. What's been happening since I last called, Jane?

Jane. Things have been going pretty well really, apart from a few small things.

CPN. That's good. Could you tell me a little more? What are the few small things that haven' t been so good?

Jane. Well we had a huge row the other night – but we've always done that anyway.

CPN. About what?

Jane. Well he said I was doing all this just to get attention, and that he was sick and tired of it – and me. But it was the only row we've had all week.

CPN. How did you feel when he said that?

Jane. Devastated. He doesn't really understand me at all, does he?

CPN. Has he done anything else to indicate how he is, or did it seem to be an outburst on its own?

Jane. He's gone very quiet. He's started working late. Or so he says. He's started to drink again.

CPN. Where do you think this is going?

Jane. Oh I don't know. It seems like I've been here before.

CPN. How do you mean?

The CPN is deliberately pacing this interaction very carefully and tentatively.

Every stage is considered. There is no rush to become sidetracked into issues such as whether or not Jane's partner 'understands' her or not. A characteristic of the tentative approach is to be constantly holding back from giving the patient the 'answer', and encouraging them to think through situations for themselves. An example of this is when the CPN asks Jane: 'Where do you think this is going?'

1.13 THE MYTH OF THE MAGIC SENTENCE

Remember that there is never a 'magic sentence' that will cure all ills and solve the patient's problem. The process of helping people can be a long and relentless process that takes time and input from many different professionals. You can make a difference to someone's experience of being ill, even if you have just started as a student. Thinking about what you are doing can only improve your helping skills. Most of what you do will be at least OK, and sometimes it will really contribute to the therapeutic process and be a positive experience for the patient.

> Margaret. I just don't know what I'm going to do. I don't seem to be able to get over what happened. These tablets aren't doing anything at all.

The natural inclination of the beginner nurse is to come up with the response that will 'make' the person feel better:

> Nurse. Keep taking the tablets – they'll start to work soon. You will get over it – be patient.

This is an example of a 'magic sentence' that is designed to provide all the reassurance that you think the person needs. However, antidepressants don't help everybody, for a range of reasons (Bloye and Davies 1999). What if Margaret *doesn't* get over it?

Here is a more thoughtful response that is not aimed at 'making the person better', but could be more useful:

> Nurse. The tablets don't suit everybody. It will be worth sticking with them though. If things don't get any better we'll arrange for Dr Roberts to see you to review them. As for getting over it, well that's more difficult. What we'll try to do while you're here is help you come to terms with what happened to you. If you can start to do that, then you might be able to pick up the threads again.

You will notice that this response is more considered, less rushed and more tentative. There are no promises or guarantees implied here but the thoughtfulness of the answer may help some people feel a little more *realistically* reassured.

1.14 SAYING THE WRONG THING

Many students are afraid of this and the possible embarrassment or shame it may bring them. It could be them that says the 'wrong thing' to a patient and suddenly they imagine that they are directly responsible for the patient bursting into tears, becoming angry, violent, or even committing suicide. Imagine the worst possible scenario:

Mary has been admitted to an acute ward three days ago. She took a large overdose of paracetamol and alcohol. Her husband was killed in a 'hit and run' accident a year ago. She left a suicide note saying: 'I cannot cope any more without him'. The student nurse is on her first day on the ward and met Mary for the first time a few minutes ago. Even though all this was mentioned in the shift handover, the student is overwhelmed by all the new and unfamiliar information and is not even sure who Mary is. She is trying to create a rapport, with the best of intentions:

> Student nurse. 'So, are you having any visitors today? Is your husband coming in?'

Mary looks stunned and then starts to sob quietly. The other patients in the day room stare at the two of them.

The student may think that she has said the wrong thing. Think of the setting, though. Mary is in a relatively safe environment where there are trained staff available to talk with her, even if not immediately. Medication could also be given to help her, if appropriate. It is likely that what has just happened in the safety of an acute ward is going to happen to Mary once she goes back to her life outside the ward. It may have already have happened, but without professional support. Here she has been *accidentally* forced to re-face the situation that may have contributed to her admission. There is help and support all around her. Outside, help and support may not be so readily available. She may have to face it alone.

It could be argued therefore that the student has said the 'right thing' in terms of helping Mary manage her grief. This does not, of course, imply that students should deliberately upset vulnerable patients with the intention of 'helping' them.

This is one way of supporting students who have made what to them might seem like a serious mistake. It is therefore very difficult, in this sense, to say the 'wrong thing' as long as the consequences are handled effectively.

1.15 NURSE OR PATIENT?

Given that most mental health nurses do not wear uniforms, it sometimes happens that patients don't know who the 'new face' on the unit/ward is, especially if a badge is not worn. This section is about how to manage the situation where mistaken identity occurs – i.e. you are mistaken for a patient/client by a patient/client. You have several options:

- *Be flattered*. Anyone can become a patient. Effective mental health nurses believe in participative/democratic care philosophies in which the symbols of control (bunches of keys on belts and authoritarian uniform styles) are seen as more destructive than constructive. So, if you look like a patient, you have been successful in getting rid of the trappings of control.
- *Be insulted*. You are likely, then, to think that mental illness couldn't happen to you and that patients are a separate type of person. How could you possibly look like one of them?
- *Be worried*. Will you have the authority to carry out your work if you look like a patient? Who else will make that mistake?

Discussion point _____

What are the pros and cons of nurses looking like patients and patients looking like nurses? How does this happen? Does it matter? Should nurses wear uniforms to stop this happening? What are the pros and cons of uniforms in mental health settings? What happens in 'therapeutic milieu' environments (Stuart and Laraia 2001)?

1.16 SELF-DISCLOSURE AND BOUNDARIES

These are another pair of related issues that sound straightforward until we start to think about the implications for us, the carers, and the recipients of our care. Much of the literature on communications, interpersonal skills and quality relationships says that self-disclosure, or telling the other person (the patient/ client in this instance) something about yourself, helps in the development of the relationship (Nelson Jones 1997, Egan 2002).

However, McLeod (1998, p. 342) suggests that 'a little self-disclosure on the part of the counsellor may be beneficial, but a lot just gets in the way'. This seems to apply whether the relationship is social or professional, but there are important differences between the two.

As a beginner in all this, be prepared for the occasional slip-up. The important thing is that you are aware that it isn't as easy as it sounds in the books. Also remember that sometimes your learning is accelerated when you make a mistake. For example, look what happens between a newly admitted patient, Patrick, and a student nurse.

> **Patrick.** Why has this happened to me? I want to go home. This place is going to make me feel even worse.
>
> **Student nurse.** I know what you mean. I think these sort of wards often do have that effect on patients.

The student nurse's response to Patrick is genuine, honest and congruent (see also section 2.11). It is the disclosing of a view or personal opinion, however, that is of little use to the patient. It could, however, be made more constructive by the skilled nurse. The intention (see also section 2.2) would be to demonstrate some understanding of Patrick's situation and try to give him some hope that others have had similar feelings but have come through it. The nurse could continue as follows.

> **Nurse.** In my experience though, most people seem to settle down after a couple of days. Give it a day or two and if it's no better we could review your whole situation with the ward team. What's bothering you at this very moment?

One of the most useful aspects of this brief interaction is that, in the single follow-up sentence, the more experienced nurse is:

- Acknowledging the patient's distress
- Offering a way forward
- Indicating a level of experience and knowledge
- Saying that the patient's experience is similar to that of others but in its own way unique
- Offering an opportunity to talk about things that are immediately troublesome.

If Patrick remains agitated, clear attempts will be made to address this further with him. In the meantime, all interventions with Patrick are aimed at monitoring his level of distress and helping him manage it. The principle here comes from techniques of crisis intervention (Aguilera 1994, Reed 1998), i.e. you acknowledge and work with the difficulty instead of turning a blind eye and hoping that it will go away.

The above example shows a professional self-disclosure in a professional setting. Things can be more difficult when dealing with personal self-disclosure in a professional setting:

Johnny. Are you married?

Nurse. No.

Johnny. How about meeting for a drink when I'm discharged?

Nurse. It's nice of you to ask, but it wouldn't be appropriate.

Johnny. Where do you live? (*Be prepared, some people will be very persistent*)

Nurse. South of the city.

Johnny. What does your boyfriend do?

Nurse. He works for a large corporation. You seem to want to know a lot about me. How come I'm so interesting? Let's spend some time talking about you?

The nurse has gradually turned the focus of the conversation back to the patient because, in the professional setting, the time usually belongs to the patient. Note that at no point has the nurse been dishonest or evasive. The response from the nurse to the probing patient has been appropriately assertive and professional, without being aggressively defensive. That, anyway, is the intention. If the patient/client is still intrusively persistent you may have to use the last resort – something like:

Nurse. It would be unprofessional of me to give my personal details to people on the ward.

The former response is, however, the preferred option as it is less of an institutionalised way to handle this admittedly difficult situation.

1.17 TIME AND TIMING

It is often disappointing for the beginner mental health nurse to find, on a new placement for the first time, that a rapport is sometimes so difficult to establish. This is even before the concept of the therapeutic relationship is considered.

Firstly, forget all about the latter until the former has been achieved. You will find that some people will warm to you quite quickly with a little bit of effort on your part. As discussed earlier in this chapter, making yourself approachable is immensely helpful at this stage. Be clear that this cannot be rushed. It takes time. The amount of time depends on your personality and the personality of each individual patient, as it is affected (or not) by their particular illness. The normally friendly, open personality may be withdrawn because of depression. The normally shy person may be over-friendly and familiar because of hypomania.

Why should patients and clients make any effort to talk to you anyway, especially if you are a student? How can you possibly be of any use to them? How can you know anything? ... and you'll be only on the ward for a few weeks anyway.

In terms of timing, again some sensitivity and a degree of empathy is needed to judge when is the right time to approach someone. Some people will talk easily to you with little prompting. Indeed you may find it overwhelming, sometimes, just how much people will disclose to you. This can be very flattering or it can be unsettling. It is sometimes to do with your accessibility as much as your approachability. As a student it is likely that you will spend more time with patients in institutional settings than the trained staff (Whittington and McLaughlin 2000).

It is important that you consider what you are going to do with all the information that patients give you in the time you have with them. It could, after all, be hours. It is essential that you make it clear, if it is not already, that things they say to you may not stop at you but will remain confidential within the care team. There is a risk that this may stop them talking to you so freely at that point, but that is preferable to you unwittingly breaching patients' confidentiality (as they may see it).

Other people will be much harder to engage with at any level. They may need a 'drip feed' approach. Each day after you have acknowledged them (they may not acknowledge you) a small gesture such as mentioning the weather, what's been on TV, whether they slept OK, or just 'How's it going?', can help to start a rapport. You may have no real expectation of a meaningful reply but at this stage even one second of eye contact can be significant. This approach will often work in terms of starting a rapport. It needs patience and persistence (see also section 2.5), as it can take weeks or months.

With some people you may never manage to get even to this point. You may try throughout the course of the placement. Your job, however, is to try with everyone and not to give up with the people who won't or don't want to talk to you. That is their right. Even the most difficult can be acknowledged each time you go to work on the placement. The job of mental health nursing needs consideration of the time you have and consideration of timing of interventions.

1.18 USE OF THE TELEPHONE

This is perhaps best avoided for a while until you feel a little more comfortable, if you are new to the placement. When you do start to feel confident enough to use the phone in a professional setting, be aware that you may be talking to someone at the other end of the line who is under stress. It may be a colleague who is trying to get extra staff for their ward. It may be a worried or concerned relative. It may be a preoccupied or impatient doctor. It may be a worried patient/client. Whoever it is, the first thing you must do is to clearly state who you are, and your status. This is so the new consultant doesn't get into a discussion about a patient before s/he realises that you don't know the patient at all. It will save you from getting very quickly and embarrassingly out of your depth. Always be polite and do not use a familiar tone with anybody unless you are absolutely certain who they are.

Gradually, as you become more familiar with the placement culture and personalities, it will be appropriate to discuss placement matters. At first, though, err on the side of caution and fetch someone who is more able to deal with things. This is a quicker way of building up a positive reputation for yourself than getting in a tangle. It is another way of acknowledging your limitations at this stage.

1.19 WHEN THE PATIENT IS AGGRESSIVE TOWARDS YOU

Try not to panic. If you don't know what to say, it might be better to leave the area quietly. Speak straight away to one of the trained staff, who may know the patient better or, if not, may have a better idea of how to manage the situation. The primary aim here is to protect yourself, so always take a conservative approach to these situations. Do not put yourself at risk, as there is never any gain, either short-term or long-term, in doing this.

   If you feel that you can contribute something constructive to the immediate situation some rudimentary skills can be useful:

- Be aware of the distance between you and the patient (or it might be a relative) – don't get too close
- Try to have a clear exit path available
- Be aware of things that might be used to hurt you … cutlery, crockery, tables, chairs, fire extinguishers, and so on (Beer *et al.* 2001)
- If you are knowingly going into a highly emotional situation, make sure that the staff know where you are
- Make sure they have heard you say where you are going
- Make sure you are under supervision and have discussed the consequences of you going into this situation
- Use steady, but not staring, eye contact
- Try to project a reasonably unflustered demeanour (but not completely calm – it can make things worse)
- *Really* listen to what the other person is saying to you
- Attempt to empathise without being patronising
- Attempt to be accepting and neutral
- Try to offer honest and realistic compromises if possible and if appropriate
- Try to avoid 'cornering' the person in any sense (Stuart and Laraia 2001, p. 635).

2 MORE COMPLEX SKILLS, TECHNIQUES AND IDEAS

This chapter looks at more ideas that can be used with most patients/clients in many settings. They are at an appropriate skill level to be attempted, under supervision, by a second-year mental health student nurse.

2.1 CONTINUALLY ASSESSING

You are always assessing. If you are aiming to be effective, as soon as you see the first patient/client of the working day you start assessing. What do they look like? How do they seem? How does this compare to your recent experiences of them? Do you need to react to this in any way?

The term 'assessing' is used in a broad sense here. Assessment skills, and the communication skills needed to do this effectively, are covered in more depth later on.

Don't forget the 'why now?' question. It has wide application in any setting and helps with assessment and history-taking.

> **Nick.** I just don't know if I can carry on any longer. It feels like the end of the road. All those years when things seemed to be going my way.
> **Nurse.** So what's significant about this point in your life? Why now?

When you are assessing, it can help to have a mini-structure to follow, in your mind. Try remembering the Acronym **HECC**:

History – What happened?
Emotions – How did they feel?
Content – What were the triggers/events/reasons?
Consequences – What happened next?

Many other sections of this book will give examples of techniques that can be used to helpfully deepen your understanding of the patients and clients you are working with.

2.2 INTENTION

This is a concept taken straight from Heron (2001). It is strongly recommended that you read the original text but the basic idea is as follows.

The effective professional carer always has an *intention* when working with patients. Heron is very specific about these:

- *Informative* – to tell patients things and 'impart new knowledge', p. 51
- *Prescriptive* – to advise, 'influence and direct the behaviour of the client', p. 40
- *Confronting/challenging* – to help patients explore other options and

'challenge the rigid and maladaptive attitudes/beliefs/actions that limit the client', p. 58

- *Catalytic* – to obtain information and to 'elicit self-discovery and learning', p. 120
- *Cathartic* – to help patients express emotions, 'abreact painful emotion, undischarged distress', p. 74
- *Supportive* – to reassure, validate, 'affirm the worth and value of clients', p. 155.

Even if you don't manage to be as clear in your intentions as Heron's categories (and you won't be, at first), it is always helpful to your patients if you have some idea of what it is you are supposed to be doing with them at any point in their treatment. If you are not clear, then take steps to obtain some clarity, such as talking to your mentor or the patient's named nurse and reading through the care plan.

Here are some examples of how the idea of having intentions can appear. Claire is sitting on her own in the day room. She is staring vacantly at a TV that is turned down very low. Her feet are tapping briskly.

> Nurse. Hi, Claire. Do you mind if I sit with you for a bit? (*Intention: Catalytic/Supportive*)
> What are you watching? (*Intention: Catalytic*)
> The volume's very low. Are you really watching TV? (*Intention: Gently Confronting*)
> So how are you feeling now it's a bit quieter on the ward? (*Intention: Cathartic*)

One of the benefits in working with focused interventions is that you can be constantly evaluating your own professional effectiveness. Did you achieve your intention, or do you need to try again using a different style of intervention? For example:

> Claire. I'm fine, thanks. I just like being on my own.

Here the nurse could accept that Claire is feeling fine. However something tells her otherwise. She tries another Cathartic intervention. Her intention remains the same – to check how Claire is feeling:

> Nurse. OK. It's just that you look rather distant, like you're not really fine at all?
> Claire. It's nothing really …. I still miss him. (*She starts to cry*)

With a combination of gentle persistence (section 2.5) and a clear intention, the nurse has been effective in *starting* to find out how Claire really is.

2.3 THE ANSWER TO THE PATIENT'S PROBLEM

It seems to be part of our human condition that we want answers to our difficulties (Watts 1987). Part of the need of some of our patients/clients is that they want to be told what to do (this is probably no different from any of us, from time to time). It is very tempting, especially at the start of a career as a mental health nurse, to want to provide answers for patients whom some of our colleagues would describe as 'needy' (Bradshaw and Haddock 1998, Estoff 1981). Like most labels in mental health, this is a relative term, as all people are needy to some degree. In the setting of mental health nursing we have to look at this concept carefully.

Discussion point

What does 'needy' mean in mental health settings? Aren't we all needy? Should we be using patronising terms like this about patients/clients? How are our needs different from those of people in mental health care?

> Veronica. I don't need this right now. How am I going to tell him that I don't want to go back?
> Nurse. That's something you'll have to think about very carefully. Perhaps we could go through some of the possible options?

What Veronica probably wants at this very moment is for the nurse to give her the answer. Perhaps what Veronica needs is someone to help her review her situation and help her with 'blind spots' (Egan 2002). The intention of the nurse could be to help Veronica discover her own answer (the Socratic approach). A problem-solving framework such as Egan's three-stage technique could be very useful here if used sensitively (see Appendix D).

Discussion point

How might a problem-solving framework look if you were to devise one yourself? How would it be different from Egan's? Does this make it more or less effective than Egan's?

> Nurse. Given the situation with Richard, and how you've described it, what do you think you really want to happen?
> Veronica. I want to be on my own again. I'm sick of his controlling behaviour.
> Nurse. So how can you start that process off? Let's go through the choices you seem to have at the moment.

Here the nurse has started to help Veronica identify some problems. It is only a start, and more might come to light. If you look at the content of Veronica's response to the nurse's question, there are at least two separate issues here. Eventually the nurse may want to help Veronica look at the two separately. At the moment, though, they may seem like the same thing in Veronica's mind.

2.4 BEING CONSISTENT

This means being professionally consistent in your behaviours, attitudes and actions. As with many other issues in mental health care, the difficulties of doing this should not be underestimated. In mental health settings you will meet people who are anything but consistent. They test the ability of any carer to the limit. The patient/client group may, because of the nature of some mental illnesses, be inconsistent. What are the benefits to the patients/clients of carers being consistent?

- Regardless of their behaviour, they find that the response is always the same or very similar. Over a period of time this will mean that negative or dysfunctional behaviour is consistently unrewarded and positive behaviour is consistently rewarded. The patient/client will experience how this feels to them.
- They experience the feeling of relative security and safety that an adult and consistent approach gives them (Berne 1975).

Given the nature of many groups, that people in groups are inconsistent in their nature, two major issues are raised in terms of mental health settings and the carers who work in them:

- Communication between carers must be encouraged to flow freely in every direction, i.e. over 24-hours among shifts and throughout the different strata of professionals.
- Differences of opinion, and even philosophies, between carers need to be addressed to reduce tensions and disparities as much as possible. This is so that a united front towards the patient or client is maintained. A divided or fragmented group of carers is not helpful to any patient (and may even exacerbate some disorders), even if individual carers think they are being helpful in their own way. This may cause friction between carers. This friction needs to be addressed if the patient or client is to be helped most effectively.

> **Nurse.** I understand the consultant said it was OK for Judith to go home at the weekend. I think that will be a disaster.
> **Ward manager.** I'm not sure. Last time she did surprisingly well.
> **Student.** I spoke to her this morning. She's very excited about it.
> **Nurse.** I told her to come back to the ward as soon as it goes pear-shaped.
> **Ward manager.** Hold on. Let's give her a chance. If she struggles, at least she's given herself an opportunity. She might learn from it. It might be better not to encourage her to race back here at the first sign of trouble.

So, here are differences of opinion that are all legitimate. The overriding issue is, which view will help the patient or client most of all? Perhaps at the moment it is the ward manager's view that will be most helpful. Two weeks ago it might have been the nurse's more conservative view that was more appropriate. As with many other aspects in mental health, the situation is dynamic.

2.5 BEING PERSISTENT

This means to 'continue firmly or obstinately' (*Concise Oxford Dictionary* 1996). Often we find the patients or clients we meet in mental health settings (often institutional ones) appear to be resistant to our interventions, despite our intention to be helpful. As is noted in several other chapters of this book, we cannot treat/help people effectively, in terms of the planned approaches we use, if we have not assessed effectively. In mental health settings the assessment process continues for the time that the person has the status of patient or client, i.e. until they are discharged to another agency, to primary care or back to their usual environment.

In order to assess accurately and effectively we may need the ability to be persistent and not to be put off by the obstacles that patients/clients seem to place in our way. Their intention, by the way, is not always to be deliberately obstructive or awkward. Sometimes the person is simply trying to gain some control over their situation. They may feel angry, aggressive, frustrated, frightened, embarrassed or uncomfortable. Look at this initial assessment:

> Nurse. How do you see yourself as ill, Darren?
> Darren. I don't. It's my parents. They're trying to get me in here.
> Nurse. What makes them feel they need to do that?
> Darren. It's because I won't do as they say.
> Nurse. What do you mean?
> Darren. They don't like me smoking and staying up all night. Can I go now?
> Nurse. Hang on. How come you stay up all night?
> Darren. I take stuff. I use the PlayStation and text people and just mess about.
> Nurse. So what do you take?
> Darren. Whizz [amphetamines]. Sometimes I have a drink.
> Nurse. How much do you take?
> Darren. Not much.
> Nurse. Your parents say that you've been having strange thoughts, that sometimes you seem very frightened. They say you won't come out of your room.
> Darren. Can I go now?

Here the nurse is using a high level of interpersonal skills, together with an attitude of interested, but gentle, persistence. If she weren't so persistent she might not get the depth of assessment data that she is on the way to obtaining. Her persistence is, of course, skilfully tempered by also being non-intrusive (see also section 1.8) when appropriate.

2.6 USING ACTIVITY

Another useful intervention is to involve the patient in activities (especially physical ones, if the opportunity can be created) that may seem to have nothing obvious to do with mental health nursing, although boredom itself is seen by some as exacerbating mental illness (Department of Health 2002a). For example, a game of Scrabble, draughts or table tennis is often accessible to nurses and patients: 'engagement in various forms of physical activities can promote therapeutic changes in the client's self concept' (O'Kane and McKenna 2002, p. 6). We can observe also how the person manages these activities and use the information in their assessment. A game of scrabble could indicate something about a person's motor skills and cognitive processes.

Activities like this can help to provide a relatively safe environment for both carer and cared for to self-disclose in a spontaneous and open way. It means that you can be genuine without needing to put on a front: 'participating staff and clients have achieved a greater level of mutual respect for each other, staff perceive themselves to be more empathic … and consider themselves more able to assist their clients and meet their needs in a more natural, caring and humane fashion' (O'Kane and McKenna 2002, p. 9).

Another possibility is to do a crossword:

Nurse. How do you do that Terry? You really seem to have a way of thinking around things.

Terry. Yeah, I was always good at these even when I was little. It passed the time. I was on my own a lot . . . .

The patient, as well as being distracted from boredom (Donati 1989, May 1995, Morrison 1996), is also reminded of what is like to be their version of 'normal', even if only for a short while. 'Activities can be a valuable therapeutic tool when they are specifically selected and aim to meet identified patient needs, but they can also be beneficial when they occur spontaneously and are diversional in nature' (Beer *et al.* 2001, p. 200).

2.7 HONESTY

This is another issue that seems straightforward but can be more complex than it at first appears. Research carried out with patients across different clinical areas, especially cancer care (Asai 1995), seems to indicate that they prefer to be told the truth. Patients receiving mental health care want us also, as carers, to be honest with them (Turnbull *et al.* 2003). In mental health settings, however, presenting the patient/client with direct honesty can sometimes generate even more difficulties for them. A considered approach has to be taken. Think about the following scenarios:

Jeremy. The doctor said she wanted me to have ECT. The gentleman who shares my dormitory said that he lost his memory when he had it.
Nurse. Yes, many people who have ECT experience that.

Jim. What does this Alzheimer's thing mean anyway? I am going to get better, aren't I?
Nurse. There isn't a cure for Alzheimer's, but there are drugs now that may slow it down.

Helen. The consultant told me I was a borderline personality disorder. What's one of those?
Nurse. It usually means someone who is difficult to be around, unstable and manipulative.

These are situations in which the nurse has given an honest response. The difficulty with this honesty is that there is a range of honest answers and the nurse has given only one of them. It is probably most helpful to the patient in the longer term to give a response that is honest but inconclusive. This is not so that we can avoid giving the answer but because in mental health care the reality of each situation often unfolds over a period of time. More open responses that are still honest, but more helpful, could be as follows:

Jeremy. The doctor said she wanted me to have ECT. The gentleman who shares my dormitory said that he lost his memory when he had it.
Nurse. There is some evidence that people do suffer from memory loss after ECT. For some it is temporary, for others it seems to be more long-term. Some don't seem to be affected at all. If you're not sure, you ought to talk to the doctor about it.

2.8 **O**PEN **DIALOGUE**

Jim. What does this Alzheimer's thing mean anyway? I am going to get better, aren't I?
Nurse. The disease means a gradual deterioration in the brain's functioning. Everyone reacts differently to this. We need to see how it's affecting you before we start coming to any conclusions about what's going to happen.

Helen. The consultant told me I was a borderline personality disorder. What's one of those?
Nurse. That term covers a very wide range of behaviours. It means many different things. You could do with asking the consultant what she meant exactly.

Another way of interpreting the above responses would be to say that the nurse, in every instance, is avoiding the issue. This is not the case. It is the closed response that is deliberately being avoided, because the truth of each situation is not yet clear. Only the passing of time will reveal it.

There are some other situations in which it seems inadvisable to be completely open. A difficulty here is that our Code of Conduct (NMC 2002) says/implies that we must always be open with our patients/clients: 'Information should be accurate, truthful and presented in such away as to make it easily understood' (p. 4). Sometimes it may seem to us that it would cause more harm than good to do this. An example is that, as professional nurses, one of our roles is to try to encourage compliance in our patients regarding the taking of medication (Stuart and Laraia 2001). Consider what might happen if you informed each patient about the full range of potential side effects of each type of medication they have been prescribed. How might they react? What might be the repercussions of this reaction for you?

Sometimes if we are not sure of how a patient might react to a piece of information we may also delay being honest. For example:

Student nurse. I'd better tell Jon that his sister doesn't want him to go home for the weekend.
Staff nurse. Leave it till tomorrow. He's not been sleeping very well and this will wind him up

Honesty can be a difficult area then, when we consider the 'interests' (NMC 2002, p. 4) of the patient.

2.8 OPEN DIALOGUE

Here, the nurse is keeping the interaction going by using 'open' dialogue. This uses words that encourage the conversation to continue, rather than encouraging it to close down, and 'is a helpful way to encourage the client's insights into his or her difficulties' (Barry 1998, p. 76). Questions are constructed that start with the words:

- What?
- When?
- How?
- Which?

47

- Why? – Note that there are some exceptions with this word. It needs to be used with care and sensitivity. Some people would see 'Why?' as being confronting and they may become defensive. This is the opposite of what you are trying to achieve. For example: 'Why did you do that?' could be experienced as a difficult and challenging question. A gentler approach could be 'What led up to you making that choice?' On the other hand, sometimes the word 'Why?' can be exactly right for some interventions when the patient/client feels relatively at ease with the material that is being discussed and less likely to feel under attack or over challenged.

Egan (2002, p. 121) suggests: 'In moderation, open-ended questions at every stage and step of the helping process help clients fill in what is missing'. All tend to encourage continuing dialogue, although they won't guarantee it. For example:

> Tony. That bloke Mel, he really winds me up.
> Nurse. It must be difficult for you. (*Closed response*)
> Tony. Yes it is.

Compare the above exchange with this one:

> Tony. That bloke Mel, he really winds me up.
> Nurse. What is it about Mel that winds you up? (*Open response*)
> Tony. It's his attitude – he's so arrogant.

Tony has had his discomfort acknowledged. He has been gently challenged to think about the implications of what he is feeling and saying.

2.9 CLARIFYING

This skill will help to deepen the assessment information you can obtain from any patient/client, and 'is most useful when parts of the client's communication are ambiguous or not easily understood' (Arnold and Boggs 2003, p. 247). It has to be used carefully and sensitively and it is driven by an almost pedantic professional curiosity. You will be surprised how often this skill reveals aspects of the patient that you otherwise might have missed. It also will show you how often you make wrong or inaccurate assumptions about the patients you work with.

Some examples of clarifying interventions are:

- 'What did you mean when you said that?'
- 'Could you just explain that again?'
- 'I don't follow you'
- 'I didn't quite catch what you just said'
- 'Could you run that past me again?'
- 'How come?'
- 'Earlier you talked about (*topic*). What were you getting at?'
- 'Sorry?'

Here is how the technique can be used (see also Watkins 2001):

> Tom. Every time we meet now, I go mad.
> Nurse. What do you mean, 'mad?'
> Tom. Well, you know, I'm angry with her – still.

Nurse. Still?

Tom. Yes. I'll never forgive her.

Here is another:

Naomi. I've got to manage this on my own. What can *you* possibly do to help?

Nurse. What sort of help do you need?

Naomi. I just want someone to make it all go away.

Nurse. How would that feel?

Naomi. Oh I don't know... (*starts to cry*).

Nurse. What's really going on, Naomi?

2.10 THE QUALITY OF THE RELATIONSHIP – WHEN IS IT 'THERAPEUTIC' AND DOES IT NEED TO BE?

Sometimes the best person to answer this question is the patient/client, although they are rarely asked. We have to make the judgement as to whether or not a relationship is therapeutic on the basis of the evidence we see, hear and feel.

The meaning of the term 'therapeutic relationship' is one that seems difficult to many students of mental health care. Perhaps to question the meaning of this term is a healthy sign in a nurse. Maybe when you *assume* that your relationships are therapeutic would be the time to be looking for the evidence.

The term 'therapeutic' is generally assumed to mean: healing/curative/making better (*Concise Oxford Dictionary* 1996). In mental health nursing, however, things are not as simple as this. For instance, some mental health nurses find themselves in the situation of being part of a care team that decides to detain a patient in hospital under a section of the Mental Health Act (1983). Legislation under discussion at the time of writing (Laurance 2003) looks as if it may increase the difficulties of some situations that nurses may find themselves working in when they have to give patients medication, without consent, outside a hospital setting. This kind of situation will really test the robustness of the therapeutic relationships between nurses and patients/clients.

It would be wrong, however, to assume that destruction of the relationship will be a natural consequence of this type of scenario. It seems to be often the case that, if enough energy and investment have gone into the establishment of a strong relationship, it may be dented but it won't sink.

> **Paddy.** There's no way you lot can keep me here. I'm going now. Don't try to stop me if you know what's good for you!
>
> **Nurse.** Paddy, you know what the situation is. I've explained it to you. I thought you understood. If you go now it will probably undo everything you've achieved since you came in, even though you've not been here very long. What is it that I've not made clear to you? Let me go through things again, and then you can decide.

Here the nurse has attempted several things with few words. She uses his first name rather than his surname. This is because at this stage she has enough investment in the relationship to do this. She then takes some responsibility for his apparent misunderstanding of the situation and the consequences of his potential action. She refers to their history of working together. She states what the consequences may be, and at the same time gives him what Berne (1975) termed a 'positive stroke'. This means a remark that is designed to help the person feel good about themselves. She again suggests that she has some responsibility in this situation and offers to try to clarify the situation. She implies that he still has some choice and he can make the choice based on clarification of the facts. She is, in this sense, trying to be empowering (see also section 2.14).

It is important to bear in mind that, if this intervention is not effective (i.e. it does not calm the situation down so that rational dialogue can continue), the patient and the staff will be entering a potentially dangerous situation. The nurse has nothing to lose, and much to gain, by trying interventions like this.

2.11 THE THERAPEUTIC RELATIONSHIP: CONGRUENCE, EMPATHY, ACCEPTANCE

Some of the signs that you *may* have a therapeutic relationship with a patient or client could be as follows:

- The patient/client feels as if they are engaging with you, even if the material/ circumstances/conditions you are trying to get through are difficult (The term 'engaging' in this setting means that they are showing some commitment to their relationship with you and with their agreed treatment plan)
- The patient acknowledges in some way that they value the relationship
- The patient seems unguarded or is willing to drop their defences a little when they are with you
- The patient is honest with you at all times, even if the truth is unpleasant
- The nurse feels a sense of loyalty
- The relationship has a sense of congruence or genuineness, about it for both parties.

A person-centred or humanistic approach to helping is usually indicated by three leading characteristics of the helper:

- Congruence
- Empathy
- Acceptance.

Congruence

This is widely considered to be a key characteristic of effective communicators (Rogers 1951). It means that you present to the outside world a person who thinks and feels the same as the one on the inside. There is no tension or difference between your outer-self and your inner-self.

Patients/clients seem to appreciate carers who are genuine and congruent in terms of their relationships with patients, colleagues and relatives. The reality of mental health nursing, however, can be a little less clear. Sometimes it is necessary to be economical with the truth (see also section 2.7). We find it necessary to withhold information from patients and relatives. We manipulate the timing of giving people information.

The reasons for this are many. We may feel, together with the care team, that these strategies are in the interests of the patient. We may be asked to do this for the same reasons. We may even sometimes make a personal decision to withhold information, on the spur of the moment. At that moment we feel ourselves to be the best judge of the situation. This last situation is best avoided, as decisions should be made by the care team.

Being always congruent, as a professional mental health nurse, is difficult. It is always, however, desirable and we should always make this 'state of being' our eventual aim with all people we meet professionally. It is important to note that in the literature the state of congruence may be known by terms such as 'genuineness, realness, openness, transparency and presence' (Nelson Jones 1997, p. 36).

Empathy

This is a little more difficult as a concept and is another idea that was brought to prominence by Rogers (1951). The nurse who is empathic (most texts use this term rather than 'empathetic') has the ability to feel some sense of the experience that the other person is talking about, and then to effectively communicate that sense. Some common and rather vague representations of this are 'being in the other person's shoes' or 'seeing the world as they see it'.

Again, things are not quite so simple as this. Many writers on this skill seem happy to leave it there. You have a sense of what the person has experienced, or you've stood in their shoes, so therefore you're empathic. The question is 'How do you know?' The only person who can make that judgement is the recipient of your attempt to empathise.

Again the value of the attempt itself should not be underrated, even if you are not accurate. It becomes real empathy when the person provides you with some evidence or clue that they recognise your empathic intervention. (Of course they are unlikely to say: 'You're really empathic'.) If you have achieved empathic accuracy they may say things like:

- 'Thanks that's really helped'
- 'At last, someone who understands'
- 'Thank you'
- 'Yes it *was* horrible/frightening/fantastic/upsetting/brilliant . . . .'

Or they may just sigh as if there has been some release, and of course there has been. The person may confirm your empathic accuracy with a non-verbal gesture such as a slackening of the shoulder muscles into a more relaxed posture. A sudden intensity in eye contact, or just a sigh of relief, or a smile, or tears welling up, may tell you that you've got it. These indicators may all be evidence that you have just been empathic. What matters here is that the person with whom you have just tried to empathise has completed the feedback loop and told you, in their own way, that you have communicated effectively.

This version of empathy is considerably more complex than the one given in many texts, but these same texts often seem to underrate the difficulties in empathising accurately. Often the impression given is that it is relatively easy. A few writers, such as Egan (2002, p. 97), indicate that this is not so: 'the truth is that few know how to put empathic understanding into words. And so sharing empathic highlights as a way of showing understanding during conversations remains an improbable event in everyday life.' They suggest that to empathise, or be empathised with, is a rare experience. Think how often you experience it in your own life.

A more structured representation of the above is the five stages of the Barrett–Lennard empathy cycle (McLeod 1998, p. 101). This, in its final stage, acknowledges the need for patient/client feedback to confirm the existence of an empathic intervention.

Discussion point

Do you think that Egan is probably right when he suggests that to be empathised with is a rare experience? When was the last time that someone empathised with you? What happened? How did it feel? What did they do/say to empathise with you? What evidence did you provide for them that they had been empathic?

Acceptance

This is the condition of being non-judgemental about the patient/client. As a professional you put on one side your views on how that person is, what they have done, how they are. You try to accept the human being and give them the respect that their status as a patient/client requires. Other terms that may be used to describe this state are 'unconditional positive regard, warmth, caring, prizing' (Nelson Jones 1997, p. 37).

This is probably one of the best examples of how the concepts of Rogers sound simple until you try to achieve them. Given the infinite range of people who work as mental health carers and the infinite range of types of people we meet in the course of our work, it is not surprising that sometimes true acceptance is extremely difficult. As professionals, though, we always aspire to this.

2.12 WHEN PATIENTS/CLIENTS SAY 'I DON'T KNOW'

When you first meet the patient/client or are in the early stages of assessment and still perhaps trying to establish some kind of rapport, small nuances of the patient's conversational style can be used by the skilled nurse to develop assessment. Many of these can slip by the beginner nurse.

The first one of these is the common phrase 'I don't know'. When you hear this phrase, it is likely to mean one of the following:

- 'I don't have that knowledge' (the phrase is therefore meant literally)
- 'I'm not sure' (because I haven't really thought about it, or I haven't come to any conclusion)
- 'I don't want to talk about it' (perhaps 'yet'? The reasons can be: too tired, can't be bothered, too intrusive, too embarrassed, too frightening, already talked about it to someone else).

The nurse can use this phrase to develop the assessment, in the following ways. With the first meaning the nurse's intervention will be to see if the unknown information is important to the patient and then to facilitate that 'education'.

The second meaning indicates that a facilitative Socratic approach might perhaps help the patient work out their own answer. The underlying philosophy here is to try to promote autonomy and independence rather than reinforcing dependence.

The third meaning is the patient saying something like: 'At this point I am unwilling to talk about this issue'. So, consider that more work is needed on the depth/quality of the relationship before this sometimes temporary impasse can be resolved. This does not mean that months of work are needed. The breakthrough may be tomorrow, or next week, given some gentle persistence.

> **Nurse.** How do you feel about visiting the residential home that Doctor Wyatt suggested might be good for you?
> **Charlie.** I don't know. (*Could mean:* 'I'm not sure at this point – I need to know more about it')
> **Nurse.** How do you think you'll get on there?
> **Charlie.** I don't know. (*Could mean:* 'I've no idea yet')
> **Nurse.** You seem a bit hesitant about all this. What's the matter?
> **Charlie.** I don't know. (*Could mean:* 'Go away and leave me alone')

If you pay close attention to the quality of the 'I don't knows' you can sometimes learn a lot about how the person is feeling/thinking.

2.13 PIGEON-HOLING DATA

Try to develop the skill of pigeon holing or compartmentalising issues in your head (this is difficult at first but do-able if you practise). You can then come back to these issues in the next few minutes, or even a week later. For example:

> **Tony.** I can't stand it on this ward any longer. The boredom is making me worse, and the other patients are getting on my nerves.
> **Nurse.** What would you really like to do? Last week you said it was good to have some space to think. Perhaps you're ready to think about going?
>
> **Naomi.** Nobody is bothered about me. I'm on my own. No one gives a shit.
> **Nurse.** Yesterday you said how well you got on with everyone at work. What's happened?
>
> **Richard.** I'm fed up with these tablets. They don't work.
> **Nurse.** When you were here last time they did seem to help you. What's different this time?
>
> **Heather.** I'm ready to go now. I don't know why you're keeping me here. I'm fine.
> **Nurse.** It's a bit soon to be saying that, isn't it, Heather? This time yesterday you were saying you wanted to die.

2.14 EMPOWERING PATIENTS AND CLIENTS

McLeod (1998, p. 109) describes empowering as 'giving people the power to change their own lives'. The term was not in common usage in mental health nursing until relatively recently but it is probably what the thoughtful and creative mental health nurse has always done.

The person who comes into contact with mental health services is potentially in a disempowered position from the moment they meet the first professional: 'Persons who are socially oppressed are often labelled as patients' (McLeod 1998, p. 257). Many things are happening to this person:

- If their friends, family, colleagues or neighbours find out, they may become the focus of remarks and ideas driven by the stigma that attaches to mental illness in our society ('Bonkers Bruno Locked Up' was a front page headline in *The Sun* in October 2003).
- As soon as they start to tell us things about themselves, they are starting to give away control to us.
- We assure them that confidentiality will be maintained within the group of professionals who are involved in their care. It is in our professional Code of Conduct (NMC 2002) but as soon as we write in the patient's notes, or discuss them with colleagues, more and more people know about that patient and confidentiality becomes more and more diluted. 'However personable, seemingly approachable or benign the person to whom we first talk might be, we have "told a confidence" to a group of people' (Dace 2003, p. 37).
- If they are being treated in an institutional setting there will be restrictions about where they can go, when they can go there, when they eat, sleep, watch TV, and so on.
- If they are being treated in a community setting, people who know them may wonder who the stranger is with them in the supermarket, or who calls once a week, stays an hour then leaves.

We can play an important role in minimising the feelings of disempowerment but we can do little to prevent them occurring altogether. What we can do is as follows:

- Try to offer choice, even in situations where patients have restricted choices (e.g. those who are detained in hospital under sections of the Mental Health Act). The creative mental health nurse will find ways to work within the restrictive parameters that mental health sections bring to the clinical situation.
- Work in a person-centred (humanistic) way. This is more likely to help the person feel valued and may contribute to reversing feelings of helplessness and slow down crumbling self-esteem for some.
- Involve the patient/client in as many aspects of their care as is feasible. Egan (2002, p. 56) suggests 'Share the helping process with clients, [they] have a right to know what they are getting into'. Ideally they should be a member of their own care team. In mental health care, this is sometimes difficult, and sometimes impossible for periods of time. It should not stop being an aim of carers, however. Barker *et al.* (2000, p. 12) suggest that 'working in an empowering way entails shifting away from exerting power of knowledge and instead collaborating with the power within the individual'.

Watkins (2001, p. 106) implies that we should be cautious about this idea: 'Empowerment may not always be an entirely positive experience for the client: some clients find the stress of choice and responsibility difficult to bear and need the support of more authoritative relationships'.

This is yet another idea that at first seems simple but can be complex to achieve in mental health settings.

2.15 THROWAWAYS

Another thing that patients/clients say that can be used to develop assessment is phrases along the lines of: 'it doesn't matter/it's nothing really'. They are often spoken in a throwaway manner, almost as if they have no value for the speaker. The opposite is sometimes true, and an interesting thing about this kind of statement is that they can mean exactly the opposite of what the person is saying. Some interpretations are therefore:

- 'It doesn't matter ' sometimes means 'It matters very much'
- 'It's nothing really' sometimes means 'It's something important'.

The effective carer is able to pick up these throwaway pieces of conversation. They can be turned into something that can sometimes dramatically increase the depth of what you know about that person and their struggles. For example:

> Nurse. Hi, Trudy, you're looking a little down this morning.
> Trudy. It's nothing really.
> Nurse. What do you mean?
> Trudy. It's just that – I'm frightened of going home. How will I manage?

or

> Nurse. Hi, Trudy, what were you trying to say in that meeting with Dr Roberts?
> Trudy. It doesn't matter.
> Nurse (*smiling*). I'm not convinced.
> Trudy. Well .... I don't think he understands me at all.

or

> Sally. Yes my treatment here has been very good . . . for the most part
> Nurse. That's reassuring, but what did you mean, 'for the most part'?
> Sally. Oh it doesn't matter, it's not important.
> Nurse. Go on, Sally, it might be.
> Sally. Well, one night I couldn't sleep, and I heard the night staff talking about me.

Sometimes, depending on the quality of your relationship, the person will disclose something really significant. Often this is only because you've gone to the trouble of acknowledging that someone may be suffering more than they are letting on, and you have been gently persistent, but not intrusive. It is important to note that sometimes, though, phrases like: 'it doesn't matter – it's nothing' are attempts to tell you to leave an issue alone.

2.16 GIVING FEEDBACK EFFECTIVELY

There is a central issue here that is important to grasp, which affects most aspects of giving and receiving feedback effectively. This central issue is *control* (Myers 1993, Barry 1998). It is important that the receiver of the feedback feels as much in control as possible. If this happens, then it is likely that the feedback has been given effectively.

Think how it feels when you are given feedback effectively. Even if the feedback isn't what you want to hear, if it is given effectively you still feel you are maintaining a sense of control over the situation. For example, if your mentor said that you didn't seem to be showing much enthusiasm during a clinical placement, ineffective feedback might leave you feeling upset, confused, defeated. Effective feedback would leave you in the position of knowing how you could remedy this, and you would be supported and encouraged when you attempted to achieve it. The meanings of effective feedback in a mental health setting can be as follows:

- The recipient (patient/client/colleague/relative) has clearly understood what you have said. There are no subtexts or hidden agendas.
- Neither the recipient nor you feels downtrodden or defeated: 'I wish I'd never brought the subject up now'.
- Neither the recipient nor you feels victorious ('I've won. That showed her').
- Delivery of quality feedback means the application of a high level of skill, involving a considerable level of empathy for the other person – even more so, if the feedback is not likely to be received favourably by the other party.

Consider the situation where you need to point out to a colleague that their attitude towards a patient is causing the patient to feel upset:

> **You.** When you talk to John like that it seems to upset him. He was telling me yesterday that he's frightened to say anything to you.
> **Colleague.** I find that very hard to believe. As far as I know I've always had a really good relationship with him.
> **You.** I think you're right up to a point, but there are some issues that he seems to find uncomfortable discussing with you. I asked him if he'd like me to mention this to you.

It may be useful at this point to consider what the effective giver of 'feedback' looks like and sounds like.

Verbal characteristics
- A steady, unemotional tone and level of delivery
- Direct ownership of the feedback: 'I think that ...' not 'It is thought that ...'.

Non-verbal characteristics
- Steady and appropriate eye contact.
- Attention given to levels and proxemics. This means that consideration is given to the distance you are away from the other person. Are you crowding them or might you seem too distant from them? Are you at a higher level than them, which might give them a feeling of being intimidated, or are you at a lower level than them, which might enhance their feelings of control?
- Attention given to timing. The above conversation between you and your colleague would need some thought as to when you said it. Straight after shift handover, just before you go home, during a break ...?

Other aspects
Attention must be given to the physical environment. For example, ensure that

the phone isn't going to interrupt, that you have some privacy, that the conversation is confidential.

As above though, the most important aspect is that throughout this interaction you attempt to maintain the other person's feeling of being in control. Thus when you are giving them feedback they don't feel crushed or humiliated (Egan (2002, p. 302) describes this as a 'personality attack').

> **Nurse.** I thought that, despite you losing your temper, you managed to bring it back enough to get your point over to your social worker. That was pretty good wasn't it? She really seems to understand your point of view now.

Instead of:

> **Nurse.** Shame you lost your temper, isn't it?

2.17 SPACE AND SILENCE

Relationships and the conversations within those relationships need space to breathe, otherwise they become suffocated. You can influence the space in your professional relationships by starting to practise talking less. This is sometimes very difficult for the beginning professional carer.

Much of the content of the first section of this book is about how you talk. This bit is about how you don't talk. As Adler and Towne (1999, p. 19) suggest: 'Sometimes there are times when no communication is the best course.' A useful technique is to give the speaker you are listening to a space of about five seconds before you start to talk. The idea is that, more often than not, you will find that the speaker has something to add to what they have just said. You will sometimes find, also, that the ideas that people 'tag on' have greater significance than the previous content. Sometimes this value is not at first apparent. Note these tag-ons and use them to help the patient. They are sometimes the result of greater processing and are added on when the person is feeling a little more secure, or a little less inhibited.

> **Jane.** I really don't think this treatment is helping me at all. If anything I feel worse, more anxious. (*The nurse silently counts...1...2...3...4...5...*) I hate myself. Why can't I even get this right?
> **Nurse.** If you look at what you've done over the last month, Jane, you'll see you've done a lot that's right.

Here, because the nurse gave Jane some space and didn't respond straight away by reacting to the issue of anxiety, the deeper issues of self-esteem and poor self-image are exposed. The nurse has been given the opportunity to work with these so she responds with an intervention that integrates both cognitive and Socratic approaches. (A cognitive approach is one where the perceptions of the patient are questioned in a supportive way, see Norman and Redfern 1997, p. 340.) She also uses the same language as Jane. If the nurse had not been silent for a very short time (although it can feel sometimes like a very long time), this opportunity to work on core difficulties might have been missed.

Try to bring more silence into your dialogue with patients. This will encourage the balance of talking to stay on the side of the patient, and the balance of listening to stay with you.

Once you have started to address this skill the next part is to be sensitive in the way you do this. Otherwise the silence that you think is productive can be viewed by the patient as exactly the opposite. Sometimes silence can become very threatening and achieve the opposite of your intention – the conversation will close down. (See also Altschuler 1997, p. 190.)

2.18 Using touch to help

This communication medium is tricky to get right but when it is used appropriately it can be very effective in terms of enhancing the rapport or therapeutic relationship: 'Whether it is a simple spontaneous gesture or a deliberate and structured activity, touch bridges the space between nurse and client, and, if it is effective, makes the nursing contact alive and meaningful' (Wright and Giddey 1993, p. 523). When it is used inappropriately, however, it can be potentially damaging.

It is difficult to explain in a book how to use this skill as so much depends on it being deployed in a spontaneous way in the 'here and now'. Here is the paradox of this intervention. It should be spontaneous in its use, yet its use needs some consideration, even if the consideration takes only a moment.

It can be used not just in situations where clients are distressed. Touch is just as valid an intervention when you are encouraging or validating. It can be used to comfort and demonstrate concern and sympathy (provided you believe that sympathy has a valid role in mental health nursing). There are issues around the acceptability of touch across cultures (McLeod 1998). Consideration should be given to when you touch, and where you touch.

- *When*. If patients/clients, relatives or colleagues are distressed, the use of touch can be supportive in their distress and validate the degree of their suffering. Similarly, it can be used to encourage positive action or discourage negative action.
- *Where*. In a professional setting there are very few places on the human body that you can legitimately touch people to offer comfort. Appropriate sites could be hands, forearms, upper-arms, shoulders.

2.19 Measuring the patient's/client's experience

This subject is also covered in Appendix A.

In mental health settings part of the job is trying to find out the worries of the patient/client in front of you. Offering a way of writing down or measuring their concern can help them explain things not only to you, but sometimes to themselves as well. Sometimes they will be very clear about what is disturbing them. Sometimes they will have no idea. You could discuss with the person the hierarchy of things that seem to be bothering them. It might then be appropriate to start using a simple problem-solving approach to start to address this, such as the Egan framework (Appendix B). The very process of helping the patient sort out this ranking can in itself be useful for them. There are many methods you can try to facilitate this:

- You could use a scale or a continuum:

Tom. I wish I knew what to do. I'm really worried about seeing my parents again after what happened last night. They think I'm completely bonkers now, don't they?

Nurse. Just how worried are you, Tom? On a scale of 1–10, if 10 is absolutely terrified, how high would you rate your fear of seeing your parents?

- You could use a pie chart (see Appendix A for examples):

  Tom. I wish I'd told my Dad what I really thought of how he is with Mum. I'm fed up with his excuses about being stressed at work. He drinks because he's just a bloody drunk.

  Nurse. If your parents' marriage could be represented by this circle (*draws on a blank sheet of paper*) how much of it is represented by them being reasonably happy and how much unhappy? Of the unhappy portion how much of that is due to his drinking? What causes the remainder of this unhappy part ?

- You could use the extreme poles of a continuum, in a different way from the above:

  Tom. I'm sure that's the reason I have so much difficulty with women. I'm just like my Dad. I didn't stand a chance, did I?

  Nurse. What's bad about being like your Dad, and what's good about being like your Dad?

- You could use a very simple stripped down genogram (see also section 2.9):

  Tom. It's no wonder he's wrecked everything again. He's played havoc in our family. Everyone's at each other's throats because of him. My sister thinks he can do no wrong. My auntie hates him.

  Nurse. I'm losing track of all these people. Does it look like this? Who else is involved? (Draws sketch on piece of paper.)

What often follows is that again the reflective process of carrying out this task brings out even more data to help you help the patient make sense of what has happened (and what is happening).

- You could ask the patient to use a diary or keep a log of events: 'The diary ... is particularly helpful in assisting the transfer of learning and insight' (McLeod 1998, p. 365).

  Tom. Every night I wake up and start thinking about the damage he's done. It seems almost deliberate. How can anyone do that? I can't work him out at all. Sometimes I could hit him.

  Nurse. Could you put a piece of paper and pen at the side of your bed? When you wake up in the middle of the night and you start thinking these thoughts, try writing them down, just as they come into your head. Perhaps next time we meet we could look at what you've written. It might start to make sense to you.

These are just a few things for you to try out when you are next talking to a patient/client in any setting and you are trying to help them sort out a tangle of conflicting ideas in their head. The main theme here is to try to turn thoughts and ideas into a visual medium. Many people find it easier to think clearly when the ideas they are struggling with are transformed into some kind of visual representation. More specialised practitioners use evidence-based measuring instruments such as the Beck Depression Inventory (Norman and Redfern 1997), the Edinburgh Post Natal Depression Scale (Spender *et al.* 2001), the Hospital Anxiety and Depression (HAD) scale (Wattis 1994) and so on, as well as their own methods of measuring patients' experiences in assessing and helping.

2.20 SUMMARIES (PARAPHRASING AND SUMMARISING)

There are two sorts of summarising: summarising at the end of an interaction and regularly doing mini-summaries as you go along. This is known in most texts as 'paraphrasing' (Adler and Towne 1999). There are many benefits of using these two similar skills, for both the carer and the patient/client:

- The patient knows you are really listening
- You can demonstrate that you understand the content of the patient's story
- The patient is given an opportunity to correct your misunderstanding of the story
- They have a chance to add something more.

Here are some examples:

Mini-summaries (paraphrasing)

Henry. At first I was glad I took the decision to retire early. It gave me a few headaches about money, though. I'd underestimated my pension contributions. It made things a bit tighter than I would have liked. That started to cause a few rows between me and Sheila. I started to see a side of her that I didn't realise was there. I could feel myself sinking gradually. I started to withdraw from her – from everybody, really.

Nurse. You felt uneasy about early retirement, it caused some rows and you started to withdraw?

Henry. Yes. And now look at the situation I'm in. Nobody phones me. Nobody calls. We don't have sex any more. We hardly ever speak. It's like I've lost her.

Nurse. So you've become very isolated?

Henry. Absolutely. I'm used to seeing people. The job I had meant that I was the centre of attention. This is very difficult. I feel lost. Where do I go from here? I can't believe I'm telling you all this. I'm used to being in control of everything.

Summarising at the end of the interaction

Nurse. Thanks for talking to me, Henry. Could I just go over what we covered to make sure I understand? The past few months have been difficult. You've found it a struggle financially since retirement. This has caused some rows between you and Sheila. She seems to have drifted away from you. You feel alone and lost, and out of control?

Henry. Yes. I don't think I can carry on. . . .

Henry is clear that the nurse has understood the essence of what he has said. He has now presented her with what is really troubling him.

Egan (2002, p. 133) states: 'Often when scattered elements are brought together, the client sees the "bigger picture" more clearly'. What has happen in the example above is that Henry has revealed that his 'bigger picture' is one of hopelessness. Now that this has been revealed the nurse is in a better position to offer help. (See also Barry 1998, p. 76.)

2.21 WRITTEN COMMUNICATION

Very early into the course there is an expectation that students start to make contributions to patient/client case notes and other related written communication such as letters to GPs and care meeting notes. All this is, of course, under the supervision of a mentor. The main principle to guide the way in which you make notes is simple, but sometimes not easy. The difficulty comes from the context in which the written communication is set. In mental health there is often a tension between how you see a patient or client subjectively and objectively. Take the patient Denise who features in Chapter 5.7. Denise is being treated in a ward setting. Her behaviour is sometimes very difficult. Many of the staff find her extremely challenging. A care note entry could read something like this:

(*Subjective*) Denise has been a real handful this morning. She was obnoxious at the breakfast table. Later on she was very irritating and was given some medication to calm her down. She slept well after that.

This report does give some impression of how Denise was over that particular time period. Some of the difficulties with it are that it gives one person's opinion of what happened. Another member of staff might not have felt irritated. They may have felt sorry for Denise because she was so frustrated about something. Also, other professionals reading this who were not present when Denise was behaving in this way might ask 'How was she a real handful? What happened? What made her behaviour obnoxious? How come she was given medication if she was only irritating? What does "slept well" mean – For a long period/ soundly/without stirring?'

There are also legal implications with all entries in care notes. Patients/clients are rightly demanding, and are being given more and more access to the notes that their carers write about them. In some instances written communications are inspected in courts of law.

Here is how the same behaviour could be described in a different and more professional way:

(*Objective*) Denise has been volatile in her mood this morning. She shouted in an abusive way at one of the other patients at breakfast time. There was no apparent provocation. Later this morning she demanded to go and would not respond constructively to repeated interventions from the staff team. She was given PRN medication as prescribed. Shortly afterwards her agitation subsided and she went to lie down. She appears to have slept from 10.30 am until time of writing. Staff continue to observe her.

This could be shown to Denise herself, if necessary (Siegler 1987, cited in

McHale and Tingle 1998). It could be shown to any other professional. It is legally credible. It is factual, non-opinionated and lacks any point of view that could not be shared by any other professional carer who was on duty that morning. Arnold and Boggs (2003 p. 599) recommend: 'be accurate, be brief, be complete'.

2.22 HOW TO FINISH

This is just as important as the way you start. Starting means addressing issues like rapport, the building of trust, the gradual acquisition of data from the patient/client, and so on. All the while, though, as you are concentrating on these aspects of care, the time is ever approaching when they will be discharged from your case load or from your ward, back to another agency, to primary care or to their own usual setting. This time should be anticipated and planned for from the time you first meet the person in a mental health care setting: 'The threads of termination are interwoven throughout the nursing process' (Arnold and Boggs 2003, p. 138).

Many patients/clients can come to experience a feeling of dependence on their carer(s) if their care is not managed thoughtfully and sensitively. Damage can be done when, at the end of their care period, that relationship is suddenly removed. This can be perceived as, or remind people of, times in their past when they have been let down, or they have let down others.

Community setting

Beryl. These shopping trips are really helping me. This time last year I couldn't even go down to the bottom of the garden. You're ever so good to me. I've not done this since my Mum died.

Student nurse. I'm really pleased for you. It's fantastic that you've done so well, especially as I leave this team next week. I'm thrilled I've seen you make so much progress.

Beryl. Next week? I didn't realise. . . .

Institutional setting

Barbara. I'm feeling so much better since those tablets started to work. You've all been very kind. I don't know how I would have coped in the flat alone.

Nurse. That's great. We'll start to sort out your discharge at the next team meeting, then.

Barbara. Discharge? Hang on. How am I going to manage? Who's going to look after me? I'll be back in here within a month – you'll see!

The finish of the relationship with a specific group of carers over a particular time is therefore indicated and sometimes negotiated very early in that period of care. In this way the patient or client always has one foot (metaphorically) back in their own setting, ready for their return to relative independence.

3 EVEN MORE ADVANCED SKILLS, TECHNIQUES AND IDEAS

These are useable in most settings for many patients/clients. The level is appropriate for the third-year mental health student nurse to attempt, under supervision.

3.1 WORKING WITH MICRO STORIES

This is a useful communication technique that most people use from time to time. Your patient/clients will all be familiar with this as most of them use this way of communicating too.

In the nurse teaching environment, the time when students invariably become most attentive is on occasions when one is telling a story. This can be about personal life experience or about some interaction with a patient, relative or other professional (maintaining confidentiality, of course). This is a form of self-disclosure. It is a feature of normal human intercourse to share experiences and give the other person our version of events as we experienced them (see also Arnold and Boggs 2003). For example:

> **Nurse.** Phil seems to be in a foul mood this morning, he swore at me when I called him for breakfast.
> **Student nurse.** The same happened to me last Monday morning, with him. Is it because he's seeing his consultant again?

In this way we share experiences to make sense of them, for us, for other people, and to gain social inclusion and a sense of belonging (Barry 1998).

The creative nurse can use this everyday phenomenon to help to engage patients and continue to sustain constructive relationships:

> **Phil.** I'm sorry I shouted at you earlier. It's the thought of seeing that Dr. Ryan again, he freaks me out.
> **Nurse.** I know what you mean. I can remember quite a few other patients who have felt like you, about Dr Ryan. He's good, though, if you give him a chance. I've known him be really helpful – he just takes a bit of getting used to.

This is a micro story that is truthful and may help to bridge the gap between the doctor and the patient. These micro stories can be expanded a little into something more substantial and helpfully significant to the patient:

> **Nurse** (*continuing the above*). I remember once we had a patient who was here for several months. She was a regular admission to the ward. She had some difficult stuff going on. At first she wouldn't even see Dr Ryan. On one occasion, though, he just caught her on a good day. After that she became quite a fan. He really helped her get sorted out, and she's not been back. If she does come in again I'm sure he'd help her just the same.

So here is a factual story that represents the doctor (or the situation) in an entirely new light to the patient. This kind of storytelling is almost always helpful to the patient and is often typical of the supportive 'behind the scenes' work that the skilled nurse can do. The technique is an important nursing intervention but has the significant advantage of being everyday and ordinary enough to not feel like a deliberate attempt to be 'therapeutic'.

3.2 STARTING TO THINK AND WORK IN AN INTEGRATED WAY

The creative, more experienced nurse is able to move across a range of techniques smoothly and seamlessly. The student will have difficulty doing this, but persistence and perspiration will pay off. The eventual aim is to be able to work in a more integrative or eclectic way. (Some of the literature does differentiate between the two terms, see McLeod 1998. However, many practitioners don't.) McLeod (1998, p. 208) suggests that the eclectic approach is where the 'best or most appropriate ideas and techniques from a range of theories or models, in order to meet the needs of the client' are chosen. Whereas the integrated approach implies 'elements from different theories and models [blended] into a new theory or model'.

Here is how an eclectic interaction may look when created by the effective nurse:

> Naomi. I'm really fed up of this place. Why isn't anybody telling me what's going on. I'm bored out of my mind? It's making me worse, and all you lot do is sit in the office.
> Nurse. What do you mean you are 'worse', Naomi?

Here the nurse is focusing straight away on the aspect that is of most importance immediately, not only to Naomi but also to her fellow patients and the nursing staff. The nurse is clarifying (see also section 2.9) the nature of what seems to be Naomi's primary concern at this moment. She is also using a catalytic intervention (Heron 2001) and working in a person-centred way (Rogers 1951). Even although you can't see it, she has paid some attention to her eye contact, tone of voice, levels and proxemics.

> Naomi. I'm getting really pissed off being stuck here. Dr Phelps said he'd see me this week. It's now Thursday and no sign of him. And anyway where's Louise (Naomi's key worker) gone? She never tells me anything either.
> Nurse. That sounds really frustrating . . . . I see what you mean. Louise is off ill at the moment. I'll bleep Dr Phelps and remind him about you.

Here the nurse is attempting to empathise (see also section 2.11). We don't know if it is effective yet. She is informing (Heron) Naomi of a new situation and reassuring (Heron) her that some action will be taken to try to remedy things. She is also creatively using a problem-solving approach (Egan 2002). Already we have seen stage 1, 'telling the story' and stage 2, 'identifying options' being used. And this is all in three short sentences.

> Naomi. Can't you tell me what's happening? I could be at work by now, getting on with my life. God knows what my colleagues must think with me being in here. There's just nothing to do.

Nurse. Let's see if Dr Phelps answers his bleep. We may get some answers then. If not I'll ask Jenny to try again this afternoon. You could give work a ring or drop them a line, to say how you're doing. Do you want some paper and a pen? How about asking some of them to visit or go out with you?

Here the nurse is again reinforcing her concern with Naomi's problems and offering a way forward. Her intention is to be supportive. She is accepting fully the frustration that Naomi is experiencing. She is not trying to fob Naomi off with excuses. These are of little interest to Naomi, who is focused on the problems 'in her face'. The nurse constantly works in a person-centred humanistic way. She has offered more options to try help Naomi with her problems.

The nurse has integrated the following approaches:

- Person-centred
- Egan's problem-solving
- Heron's intervention analysis
- Appropriate interpersonal skills.

She will probably apply this cluster or group of skills to help many patients and clients.

You will find that thinking and working in an integrated or eclectic way is difficult at first. To start to do this it is probably most realistic to reflect on your recent effective interventions with patients. This could be done in supervision, with a colleague or on your own. Is it possible to separate out the component parts of the interaction into different theories or approaches? Which ones worked most effectively for this patient? Why was that? Which ones do you like best or find most useful? Whatever range of approaches you use, the important thing is that you are thinking what you are doing and are better equipped to be able to explain, and justify, your rationale and/or evidence base.

Discussion point

What are the pros and cons of working in an integrated way? How is this different from working eclectically? What's wrong with making it up as you go along? Wouldn't it be better to stick to just one approach or theory?

3.3 PROFESSIONAL ASSERTIVENESS

The traditional literature on this area tends to focus on aspects such as posture, eye contact, your 'rights' and so on. As in other parts of this book, I will try to present a real life view of what it is, why you sometimes need to do it, how it feels and the results you may obtain when trying to be assertive in a professional setting.

Firstly, it is important to note that many of the core skills that make you socially effective as an assertive person will make you professionally effective as an assertive nurse. These core skills are as follows:

- Being clear about what it is you want/need
- Having a 'Plan B' – i.e. what if you can't get it?

- Being prepared to negotiate/compromise
- Being clear that this isn't about winning, it's about obtaining a reasonable result (of course the term 'reasonable' has many different meanings!)
- Using appropriate interpersonal skills, i.e. being aware of your: eye contact, voice tone, posture, distance from the other person, difference in levels between you and the other person, and so on
- Being aware of the fine line between the right level of assertiveness for that situation and the wrong level of aggression
- Being aware that your gender may be an issue here – some assertive women will be seen as aggressive women by some men, almost regardless of how skilful they are. Also, according to Arnold and Boggs (2003, p. 370): 'Many nurses, especially women, have been socialised to act passively'
- Realising that in some situations you will be good at it, and in others you won't
- Realising that this 'rule' applies to everybody – no one is consistently assertive.

There are some differences between social assertiveness and professional assertiveness. The key issue is that in social situations what may be at stake is the imbalance between what you want from your supermarket/garage/restaurant/clothes shop and what you have got, or are getting. In the professional setting the patients' care is always the issue, even if sometimes the link is not obvious.

Whether or not the setting is social or professional, the seed of every need to be assertive is some manifestation of conflict, either actual or potential. As conflict is an unavoidable part of our lives, it follows that, to constructively resolve some of these conflicts, the issue of personal and professional assertiveness deserves some attention. It is not just a 'bolt-on extra'. It could mean the difference between you staying in the job, feeling satisfied and fulfilled, and leaving the job feeling undervalued and over-run. It could mean the difference between flourishing and surviving: 'How are nurses going to be supported to take on new roles and responsibilities when they can't even take a meal break, let alone a study day?' (Malone 2003, p. 1).

Here are some examples of how professional assertiveness could look.

> **A staff nurse.** Nip and make us all a tray of tea will you? The consultant has black coffee, by the way ... no sugar.
> **You.** I'm in the middle of a discussion with Mrs James (*a patient*). I need to stay with her. Could you get someone else to do it? When I've finished with her I'll sort out the tea then.

You have not refused, regardless of your feeling about making tea for everyone. (Don't forget, this gesture is a great social lubricant when you are new at a placement.) You have put the needs of a patient first. You have offered the compromise of a tray of tea later on, if it has not been provided by then anyway.

> **A doctor.** Could you get me a sphyg. – and get me this patient's notes while you're at it, will you?
> **You.** I'll sort out Mrs James's notes. You'll find the sphyg. in the cupboard over there.

Again, you have compromised, and you have shown more respect to the patient than the doctor has. The distribution of tasks is renegotiated by you. This is an important habit to get into. You may be working with this doctor again as a qualified nurse. Your relationships with other professionals start to form when you are a student.

> **A relative.** Could you pack my husband's bags for me? We're going this afternoon.
> **You.** I'll show you to his room so you can make a start. I'll join you in a bit just to sort out the final details.

You have again not refused, you've just made it clear that your role in this is slightly different. You may, by the way, sometimes prefer to help with tasks like this. You can learn a lot about people doing these mundane jobs with them.

> **A patient.** It's OK if my girlfriend takes me to her place for the weekend, isn't it? I'll be all right.
> **You.** Well, you need to check it out with the nurse in charge. I'll ask him to talk to you about it.

A clear example of passing on the responsibility for this situation quickly and professionally. You make sure that you do what you say you are going to do. This will avoid any future misunderstanding. (See also Jacobson and Jacobson 1996, Gelder 1999, Stuart and Laraia 2001.)

3.4 THE IDEA OF PSYCHOLOGICAL CONTAINMENT

This means the psychological 'holding' of a patient/client or 'the management of another person's difficult feelings which are otherwise uncontained' (Casement 1994, p. 132; see also Wright and Giddey 1993). It is nothing to do with sections of the Mental Health Act or locked ward doors. Containment, in this context, has the same positive feel to it as does 'asylum' when applied to a place of safety. The sense of containment should feel the same for the recipient.

Using interpersonal skills, the nurse team can create a sense of containment for a patient/client. It is difficult for an individual nurse to provide a sense of containment in an institutional setting; however, individual carers often try to do this outside these settings. This would be attempted in the clear understanding that this sense is temporary and that dependence on the providers of the containment is a risk of this strategy.

> **Michael.** I feel like I'm going to explode. I hate myself. The crap person in my family was always me. When I cut myself it feels like the pressure goes.
> **Nurse.** It sounds really horrible for you. You know that we'll try to discourage you from cutting. Sometimes we won't be successful and you'll do it anyway. But try to talk to one of us first. We'll try to help you through this.

Here the nurse has tried to empathise by saying to Michael words that try to capture and empathise with the agony that he sometimes experiences. She has given him no authoritative guarantee that he will be stopped from self-harming. She has tried to assure him that someone will be available for him to talk to, if he chooses this option. She has implied that other options will be explored that may help him as much as, or more than, cutting. This would always be a nursing intention anyway. She tries to help Michael feel 'held' or 'contained' to foster a feeling of safety and security within Michael.

3.5 The observe/assess/react cycle

This is another essential tool in the repertoire of the effective mental health nurse. It is one of the things that can make the job of the mental health nurse so tiring when it is done properly. This doesn't take into account any physical interventions that the nurse may need to make, such as assisting with bathing, dressing, feeding patients, and so on, depending on the care setting.

What the effective nurse will be doing is observing, in both a generalised and a more focused way, everything that a group and some individual patients are doing. This skill is developed over time until it is carried out almost subconsciously. The experienced nurse develops a sophisticated selective perception whereby superfluous information is filtered out and important information is kept on hold or processed.

Discussion point

What makes some patient information superfluous? On what basis do we make that kind of judgement? What could be the consequences of us making misjudgements?

This is the 'assess' stage. The nurse is trying to make sense of what s/he has seen, heard, touched, smelled and intuited, set against the background of the needs of that patient as perceived by the care team. Based on this, the nurse then reacts. The nurse may approach the patient, approach a colleague, write in the care plan, involve a relative or do nothing, apart from consciously registering some change. Here are some examples of how this might happen.

Institutional setting
Maxine, a 19-year-old girl, has been on the ward for three days. She presents as very quiet. She keeps herself to herself. She is observed by Jo, a staff nurse, as looking preoccupied this morning. She is staring into the middle distance and rocking gently. Her hands are twisted tightly together. Jo assesses.

Jo. Hi, Maxine. You're looking a bit on edge this morning. What's happening?
Maxine. I can't take any more of this place. I want to go home

Jo reacts.

Jo. Can I sit with you for a minute? So what's getting to you?

Community setting
Derek, a 50-year-old divorced man, is being visited by Louise, a community psychiatric nurse. She observes that he seems more relaxed today than usual. Previously he has been tense and quite agitated. She assesses:

Louise. You seem a bit more at ease today. Usually you're really on edge when I'm here. What's happened?

Derek. Oh, nothing, really. I've just been doing a lot of thinking and I've come to a decision.

Louise suddenly feels uncomfortable. She assesses some more:

Louise. I get the feeling you're thinking much more than you're telling me here.
Derek. I've decided there's no point any more.

Louise reacts:

Louise. What do you mean, no point any more?

Day unit setting

Edna, an 80-year-old widow, attends the day hospital twice a week. Ashok, a staff nurse, observes that Edna seems very confused and disorientated today. Usually she is OK once she has been there for about half an hour. Today, something is different. He assesses:

Ashok. Morning, Edna. Did you have a good weekend?
Edna. The trees need pruning. I'm just off to get the shears. Watch the cat will you?

Ashok reacts to the feeling in the content, rather than the content itself (this is a validating approach – see Norman and Redfern 1997). After all, Edna has lived in a city-centre care home for the last two years. She doesn't have any trees or a cat.

Ashok. You seem a bit busy and rushed today, Edna.
Edna. Yes, lots to do, lots to do. – See you later.

3.6 'The problem is …'

When you hear a colleague or a patient or client say these words try adding an 's' to the word problem and changing the 'is' to 'are'. In the context of mental health nursing (and most other settings) very few problems are solitary in nature. Most difficult situations seem to have several problems that are dependent on each other or that interconnect. Sometimes the interconnections are not at first apparent. A skill of the nurse is to spot them, make sense of them and use them to help the patient.

Solving just one difficulty often isn't the whole answer and doesn't make the other problems disappear. The opposite is sometimes the case – resolution of one problem often means exacerbation of another.

A common problem experienced by many sufferers of mental ill health is that, however successful their treatment is in terms of stabilising behaviour and so on, their fate is often to return back to the destabilising conditions that triggered off the episode in the first place. Hence their problem does not exist in isolation. It is connected to other factors.

Also, as an effective psychiatric nurse, you will be aware that the nature of the problem changes depending on who is looking at it. For example:

Nurse. The problem is Tom's mother. She doesn't seem to want to let him go.
Tom. The problem is I'm scared to leave home. I know the staff think that Mum is interfering, but look what happened to me last time.

Tom's Mum. The problem is that nobody knows what Tom is really like at home. He can't manage on his own.

Tom's Psychiatrist. The problem is that Tom has become over-dependent on his mother

So, a possible resolution of this is to try and facilitate a network of communication to start to work towards a consensus view of the range of problems in this situation. Often the mental health nurse is well placed to start this process off.

3.7 USING IMAGES AND IMAGERY

It is often very useful to try use images in your language with patients/clients as a more effective way of communicating. Using images can help people tune in quickly to what you are trying to say, or alternatively can help you tune into what a client is trying to say. For example:

Nurse. Your decision to discharge yourself has turned into a bit of a cliffhanger again hasn't it?

Peter. How do you mean?

Nurse. Your wife is afraid that you might topple over the edge again if you go home now.

Peter. I'll be OK. I'll keep well away from the edge this time. If I start to slide I'll call you or come back ... I promise.

Here is another:

Nurse. You're seem to be trying to do too much too quickly. You're trying to reach the finish before you've checked your brakes. How are you going to stop?

Daniel. It feels like the finish is a long way off and the accelerator won't work properly. I don't care about the brakes anyway.

Nurse. Does this remind you of last time, though?

And another:

Sophie. It feels like a black cloud is hanging over me

Nurse. What would make the black cloud go away?

Nelson Jones (1997) also discusses extensively how imagery can be used in a range of therapeutic settings and suggests that in a setting where a cognitive approach is used the technique is useful for rapidly accessing 'automatic thoughts'.

3.8 EVERYTHING BEFORE THE 'BUT'

This is another everyday speech pattern that most people use. It can help you access what people really think about the situations they are in:

Joan. My named nurse is very nice and she means well *but* I don't think she really understands where I'm coming from.

Staff nurse. Student nurse Cooper is always professional *but* I wish she'd take her time more and not rush into conclusions about people.

Doctor. John's family are interfering, I agree, *but* at least they are trying to help.

This has an everyday application. Listen for the words after the 'but'. There you will hear the truth *for that person*. The words before the 'but' were dismissed by Fritz Perls (a contemporary of Rogers) as part of his 'hostile stance to over-intellectualisation' – 'Everything before the BUT is bullshit' (McLeod 2003, p. 162).

As with many of the other assessment ideas in this book, the importance of this one is that it has everyday ordinariness and therefore everyday application.

3.9 Genograms

These are another useful tool for any mental health nurse: 'a genogram is not only a method for gathering information, but an intervention in itself' (McLeod 2003, p. 118); 'a succinct way of organising family history [that] can highlight patterns and themes that have recurred through successive generations and are influencing the present' (Watkins 2001, p. 131). They have wide application and can be used in many situations.

Jean has been feeling very low in mood for several months. She has recently started to have panic attacks. She no longer goes out. Her teenage son does all the family shopping. Jean's daughter refuses to help and tells her to 'snap out of it'. Jean has recently been referred by her GP to a community psychiatric nurse, who assesses her.

The nurse uses a diagram of the family organisation to help in Jean's assessment. Jean mentioned a half-brother as she was talking about her past life to the nurse. She became a little bit upset. The nurse starts to sketch out the family system on a piece of paper with a pencil. She draws a symbolic sketch of Jean's parents and their relationship (they divorced), then representations of Jean and her late twin sister:

Nurse. So, you talked about your twin sister who died. How did the half-brother fit in? Could you show me?

Jean. He didn't fit in. I don't know much about him. I only found out accidentally. Mum was in a rage one day and she told me. He was because of Dad's affair with Auntie Fran before they divorced.

Nurse. So what happened to him?

Jean. Apparently he died in a road accident. I wish they'd have told me. I always wanted a brother.

Nurse. It strikes me looking at this [genogram], that you've had a lot of loss in your life.

Jean. Yes. I'm terrified it's going to happen to me again. I don't know what I'd do if anything happened to the kids.

Nurse. How old are they, Jean?

Jean. Leanne is eighteen, Jack is fifteen. I'm on my own with them since I divorced Harry.

The nurse then adds symbols for Jean's children and notes that Jean too, is divorced.

Wright and Giddey (1993, p. 69) talk about an interesting version of this: 'Virginia Satir, one of the early family therapists, likens the family to a mobile. If you touch a mobile, you can observe the sequence of movements that occur.

Genogram of Jean's family relationships sketched out by the nurse

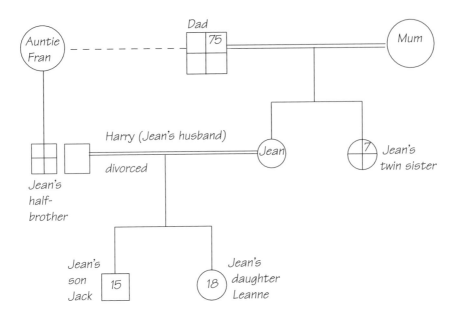

Parts of the mobile are affected differently depending on how they are connected to each other.'

See also Arnold and Boggs (2003) for more in depth discussion of genograms.

3.10 DIFFERENT LOSSES

As a beginner, you will find that sometimes a useful question to ask yourself (and of course, when it's appropriate, the patient/client) is: 'Where do losses fit into this person's life?'

The obvious big loss that all of us have to face is the death of someone close to us or someone who has been significant in our life for some reason. Most people handle, or manage or cope with this kind of loss in their own way, and get through it. Many of these losses we do not 'get over'. Rather, we learn to live with the loss and it becomes part of our history.

Some people you meet in the course of your work will be having difficulty coming to terms with their loss(es). The literature suggests that humans in Western society grieve in a particular way (Gelder *et al.* 1999, Norman and Redfern 1997, Stuart and Laraia 2001), although a contemporary view at the time of writing seems to suggest that to be too formulaic about the application of these models is mistaken and inappropriate (Jacobson and Jacobson 1996).

There are many things to take into account here, though, for the thoughtful mental health nurse. First, be careful about the assumptions you make when trying to understand and support people in your care who have had a significant loss and who are trying to manage the situation. For example, Tom is very low in mood since the death of his mother. She died after a short illness about two years ago. It is the anniversary of her death in a week's time. (Anniversaries of the death, birthdays and the first Christmas may be difficult to cope with – Jacobson and Jacobson 1996, Worden 1988, cited in Gibson 1991.)

> **Tom.** I hate this time of year. It all comes back again. I can't get it out of my head – it's like drilling through my brain.
>
> **Nurse.** Sounds like it's still really hurting you. What's the worst thing about it for you, Tom?
>
> **Tom.** We had a row about my Dad just before she died. I was sticking up for him. She had no right to be so horrible about him. I wanted to say that, but I was too scared of her ... always was. Now I feel that I can't finish the situation with either Dad or Mum. I'm not sorry she's dead, I just want to tell her how I feel. I never could, and now I never can. That's typical of me. Just like Mum said to me, I'm useless.

It is easy to always assume that people are upset about the loss, but it could be something very different. Tom actually says that he is not sorry that his Mum is dead. He is sorry about the opportunity he has missed, and perhaps also sorry that there seems to be no way out of the pattern that has been established in his early relationship with his mother.

Beware of assuming that people react the same as you to major loss. Even people's perception of what constitutes major loss can be very different. Tentatively use your rudimentary skills to explore the territory first. As in the example above, just a few sentences can produce so much potentially useful data for the nurse to really help the patient that it is sometimes difficult to know where to start.

3.11 WHEN THE PATIENT FINDS THE NURSE ATTRACTIVE (AND *VICE VERSA*)

This can happen in any professional nursing setting (Clarke 1999). It is not exclusive to mental health (McLeod 1998) but the difficulties arising from this can be more complex in this branch of nursing because of the sometimes intense nature of the relationship that can develop between nurse and patient/client (Watkins 2001).

If the patient/client is giving you signals that they find you attractive, it might be helpful to understand some of the reasons for this, so that you can work out how best to manage it.

Many people who are in mental health care will be in crisis or a period of difficult transition. They may be feeling out of control or as if control has left their life. Myers (1993, p. 113) discusses the significance of control: 'having a strong sense of controlling one's life is a more dependable predictor of positive feelings of well being'. They are likely to be feeling isolated or alone (Watkins 2001) Then into their life comes a person who is willing to listen to them and give them attention. The significance of this should not be underestimated. Think about the last time someone actually sat down with you and really listened to you, without adding their own agenda to the conversation. (This is also discussed earlier in section 1.1.) Add to this set of circumstances that for whatever reason the person also finds your personality or physical appearance attractive, and you may have a complex set of issues to deal with.

Nurses who work using an understanding of the psychodynamic approach would suggest that in this situation a phenomenon called 'transference' is affecting the relationship and that this needs to be handled with care and thoughtfulness. The psychodynamic approach puts great emphasis on the significance of human relationships, especially early-life relationships such as parenting figures, and the effects that this has on us as adults (see also Chapter 2). An explanation of transference would be that subconsciously you are reminding the patient of someone from their past life who affected them in some significant way. They may have felt a strong emotion for this person. Now you are the focus of that emotion, or at least something that is beyond the usual meaning of the carer/patient relationship.

The way you handle the early sessions or interventions with this person can set the tone for the rest of your relationship. It can make things productive and clear, or difficult and confusing for both of you. The effects can also spill over into the dynamics between you, some of your colleagues and some of your patients. Consider the following:

> **Calvin.** It feels like you really understand me. No one's ever taken much notice of me before. We get on really well, don't we? It's like I've known you forever. When I'm discharged, could we meet up perhaps?
> **Nurse.** I suppose when you're discharged it wouldn't do any harm. But I can't do anything while you're a patient. We're not allowed.

Here the nurse, in just three sentences, has:

- Been ambivalent – is Calvin clear whether she does or doesn't want to see him?
- Put the responsibility for her actions on to the organisation
- Implied that she agrees with his view of the situation – that they do get on really well and it is like they've known each other for ever.

Here the nurse has a potentially even more difficult situation to withdraw from than it was already. It is impossible to forecast what might happen if she did choose to see Calvin after he is discharged. What is easy to forecast is that the perceptions within the relationship are likely to change. Calvin may find out that the nurse doesn't actually understand him so well on a non-professional basis. They may find out that sometimes they don't get on so well. What might happen if he becomes unwell again and needs re-admission? It would seem that, in these situations, the most caring course of action is something like this:

> **Calvin.** It feels like you really understand me. No one's ever taken much notice of me before. We get on really well, don't we? It's like I've known you for ever. When I'm discharged, could we meet up perhaps?
> **Nurse.** That's nice of you to say that. In some ways I think I do understand you. It's good that we get on. Things will change when you go home, and our job here is to help you get towards that point.

Here the nurse has acknowledged Calvin's feelings towards her. She has responded in a way that owns her views. She has indicated that the relationship has a 'sell-by date' and that her behaviour towards Calvin is part of her professional role. There is no ambivalence here. She has tried to make the nature of their relationship clear. This is a very caring action and puts the needs of the patient first, even though Calvin, at this stage, may not see it this way.

In addition, Egan (2002, p. 213) suggests that a skill to use in situations like this could be 'immediacy', or 'What's going between you and me right now?' The continuation of the nurse's response to Calvin, using this skill, could be:

> **Nurse.** I wonder what has happened here to cause you to say those things about me?

Sometimes in the course of your work you may meet patients/clients whom you find attractive. Again, it is useful to understand some of the processes that may be happening. In all nurse–patient relationships the balance of power, and thus the potential to abuse this power, lies with the nurse. The nurse is always part of a team. Decisions about the treatment of patients are made by these teams. Ideally the patient is involved with this decision making process (Altschuler 1997) but, with the best intentions, sometimes this doesn't happen. If you have a degree of empathy for a patient/client who seems to be in an isolated situation, this can change into a kind of protectiveness. Sometimes this can produce very strong feelings. If this is combined with an attraction for the person's physical appearance or personality, a difficult set of issues is again raised.

As above, the psychodynamic approach would suggest that here strong counter-transferences are affecting the relationship. Something in the patient is triggering off past memories or responses for you, although you may not even realise it. There are several ways of managing this, and it *must* be managed, as the implications of a non-professional relationship with a patient in care are extremely serious and may ultimately mean the loss of your job.

- Be very careful about the intervention style you use with the patient. As indicated above, you must be absolutely clear in your own mind that the nature of your relationship is to help the person in care to recover and leave the care setting. This is probably the best thing that you can do for this person, and it is truly caring. Therefore, your interventions are free of ambivalence in your own mind. Everything you do or say is set in the context of your professional work. There is no leakage into the fantasy world of 'How it might be'.
- If you feel safe to do so, a constructive way to manage this situation would be to seek clinical supervision. It goes without saying that you would need a high level of confidence in your supervisor to broach a topic like this. As a beginner your supervisor is likely to be your assessor, so again, the difficulties for you in this situation are not to be underestimated.
- Remind yourself of the seriousness of the implications of not being clear. This could mean the end of your career at worst. (See also Stuart and Laraia 2001.)

3.12 USING THE TRAY OF TEA

You make a tray of tea for a group of patients in the day room. Of course, you check that this is not a dangerous action, as it might be, for example, if you are working in a setting where the cups may be thrown around and used as weapons. Assuming that all is safe on this front, the tray of tea is yet another medium that can be used by you on several levels.

- It is an empowerer. You have made the tea for the patients, and therefore you are not putting yourself in any position of authority. You have done a group of people a favour or a kindness.
- It is another method of developing assessment. Who offers to pour? How is this accepted and acknowledged? Do people help themselves? Who needs to be helped? Who manipulates help for themselves? Who has several cups? Does anyone notice this? Is the group split? How is it split? Do people work democratically or as individuals who are just concerned with themselves? Does the social tradition of the tea tray trigger off 'normal' behaviours in people who have been seen as 'not normal'? For example does the withdrawn and depressed lady manage to get her own drink, or does the more active lady who sits with her do it for her? Do you intervene and prompt the withdrawn lady with an invitation to 'join us?'
- It can help to develop normal social habits in an abnormal social setting. It can help to maintain respect for other people's space and personal habits. These are the very things that tend to be eroded in institutional settings.

Above is an example of how the tray of tea can be used to help you help others in institutional settings, by deepening your assessment data. Try to think of other methods of using the same principles as above. For example working out a rota with a group of people as to who will fetch sweets and crisps or newspapers. It would be interesting to see who leads and who follows. Does the withdrawn lady mentioned earlier respond to this? Here is an opportunity to assess how her treatment is working if you approach her with this task every day. This approach could even be part of her plan of care.

3.13 CULTURAL DIVERSITY

This book has been written by a white, middle-class man. Whether I like it or not, the values that connect to this position in our society will have influenced the content. Using the rudimentary skills described earlier it is feasible that you will be able to make some connection with most people, almost regardless of their age, gender and current mental health condition. However, if you are using these skills with a culturally or ethnically different person who is perceived by our predominantly white society to have a mental illness, a different range of problems may arise.

What are the difficulties if they don't understand your verbal language and you don't understand theirs? Resolving this is not as easy as just finding an interpreter, as there are widely recognised problems with this (Lago 1997), although of course it may help. McLeod (1998, p. 174) recognises the difficulties that can arise from 'subjective culture': 'it is much harder for someone who does not share the same subjective culture to appreciate the meaning or implications of the words used by a client'. This is an issue that warrants serious consideration, given the significant contemporary increase in ethnic and cultural diversity in our society: 'There has been an explosion of literature on diversity and multiculturalism over the last few years' (Egan 2002, p. 49).

This is not a new issue and it does not necessarily refer to white/black diversity. There are issues here about ethnicity, class and gender. The author has witnessed on many occasions white, middle-class psychiatrists demonstrating a complete lack of empathy for, and understanding of, a range of white people. A similar situation can occur when a psychiatrist from an ethnic minority tries to understand the story of a patient/client from the ethnic majority.

The thoughtful mental health carer will experience increased difficulties in connecting *meaningfully* with patients/clients if their cultural/ethnic background is different from his/her own (Lago 1997). Some cultures do not even recognise mental illness in the same way as the West: '... mental illness is unrecognised by traditional Chinese medicine. For example, a Chinese equivalent term for depression does not exist' (Barraclough 2003, p. 18).

There is no easy answer to this problem. It is important to remember that just because the person who needs your help cannot understand your verbal communication it does not mean that you are paralysed as a helper. The basic non-verbal skills such as acknowledgement of people, respect, a smile, considered eye contact, and even careful use of touch (see also section 2.18), can still make a helpful impact on a difficult situation, although Lago (1997) warns of difficulties with even these approaches in some cultures.

There is some evidence that unsophisticated and simple conditions can improve the experience of the patient who is in an environment that is alien to them. Some interviewed patients of an ethnic minority said: 'the three best things (were) being able to talk to someone, some staff attitudes, being in a calming environment and hospital foods' (Sathyamoorthy 2001, p. 18). All except the first of these can be achieved, at least in part, without necessarily understanding the other person's verbal language. The creative nurse will use all resources available. Maybe a colleague from a similar cultural/ethnic background could help. A member of the patient's family may also be able to assist, especially if they are from a culture that is based on 'kinship systems' (Lago 1997).

Historically, many patients in mental health settings who were of ethnic minority or culturally different backgrounds were to all intents and purposes ignored or given minimal input of a medical model type. 'Sadly, for some ethnic minority groups the lack of adequate cultural knowledge within nursing prevents proper interactions taking place in any meaningful way' (Cooper, cited in Wright and Giddey 1993, p. 191). Also some writers suggest that a 'double discrimination' will be suffered (Raleigh, cited in Kaye and Lingiah 2000, p. 29).

Consideration of more creative approaches are likely to make a difference to the patient. At least they may appreciate that efforts are being made. Also, as Egan (2002, p. 51) says, 'Your clients are individuals, not cultures, subcultures or groups. Remember that category traits can destroy understanding as well as facilitate it.'

This whole area does not have any easy answers and it is an issue that will not go away. As a nurse in this setting you have to do the best you can with what you have. In many areas the resources and even the willingness to do this may be limited.

3.14 SUICIDE

You may encounter suicide early in your training, or it may not happen until you are qualified, but if you stay in the job of being a mental health nurse it will happen. Reading about it in this book cannot prepare you for the event. You may be very surprised at the feelings you experience and the feelings you see being expressed by your colleagues. A range of some of your and your colleagues' possible responses to this event could be as follows:

- *Guilt*. 'Why didn't I/we see that coming? Could I/we have done something more to prevent it?'
- *Relief*. 'They were having a miserable time. Perhaps it's the best thing for them.'
- *Anger*. 'How could they do this? What about the people they've left behind?'
- *Resentment*. 'It was a coward's way out.'
- *Ambivalence*. 'It doesn't really bother me.'
- *Shock*. 'I can't believe it!'
- *Acceptance*. 'It's bound to happen sometimes in this job.'
- *Questioning*. 'How could we have stopped it happening? How do we prevent it happening again?'
- *Defensiveness*. 'It wasn't my/our fault. We/I did nothing wrong.'
- *Resignation*. 'I don't know what else we could have done.'
- *Fear*. 'There's going to be a witch hunt about this!'

Whatever the response(s) are, it is necessary for the staff involved in the care of the patient, including all shifts and grades, to participate in a debriefing (see also section 6.11). This will provide a supportive environment for carers to start to come to terms with, and perhaps have a forum to discuss, their feelings about what will always be a feature of mental health care.

4 DISORDER-FOCUSED INTERVENTIONS

This chapter attempts to show how the skills/techniques/ideas described in Chapters 1–3 can be used to try to help adult people with a range of mental health disorders. The structure of the chapter has been designed to reflect the disorders described in contemporary mental health literature, and more specifically the 'Changing Minds' campaign (Royal College of Psychiatrists 2002). The group known as 'complex needs' (Keene 2001, Beer et al. 2001) is addressed in Chapter 5.

The intention is to demonstrate that often there isn't much difference, if any, in the way we initially approach any of these people in terms of the basic skills/techniques needed to do this professionally and effectively. These interventions are aimed at the beginner who wishes first to create a rapport and then to develop it a little further, in conjunction with any care plan, during both the initial assessment stage and later on. It is not intended for specialists, although there may be material here that is of interest and use to specialists, especially those who are assessing or mentoring mental health students of any profession. The interventions described are not intended to be prescriptions of how it should be. They are starting points for considered discussion and/or reflection as to how interventions could be.

I acknowledge that sometimes it is not helpful to describe mental illness as a list of symptoms. Mental illness is sometimes more chaotic and complex in its nature. This will be acknowledged and addressed to a greater extent in Chapter 5.

4.1 PEOPLE WITH ABNORMAL PERCEPTIONS

Introduction

People with abnormal perceptions may be regarded as having psychotic illness, suffering with schizophrenia or being schizophrenic. Schizophrenia describes a range of mental disorder that affects the lives of around 1% of the population in the Western world. This statistic seems to have been consistently quoted over a period of many years. The disorder shows itself in terms of 'problems of thinking, feeling and behaviour of sufficient magnitude, to cause severe handicaps in virtually every area of living. This population suffers a miserable quality of life' (Gournay 2003, p. 14).

The signs and symptoms of the disorder are often categorised into two broad groups – negative and positive symptoms. Positive symptoms are hallucinations, paranoia, delusions and bizarre behaviour. These signs are often referred to as 'florid psychotic symptoms' (Varcarolis 1998, p. 627) and are often easy to see. Less easy to spot straight away are the negative symptoms. These are apathy, lack of motivation, anhedonia (inability to enjoy things) and poor thought processing: '[these symptoms] persist and seem more fundamental' (Varcarolis 1998, p. 629).

It has again been consistently noted over many years that a high percentage of people who suffer from this disorder seem to inhabit lower socioeconomic groups. 'This has been attributed to social disorganisation and social stresses as well as to evidence that some people in a prepsychotic phase drift down the social scale' (Berkow *et al.* 1992, cited in Varcarolis 1998, p. 627).

It would appear that the positive symptoms respond quite well to nursing and medical interventions such as medication, pre-emptive nursing responses such as monitoring prodromal symptoms (the signs that the person is going into relapse) and family support. Unfortunately, the negative symptoms seem to be more resistant. 'The positive symptoms ... are the least important prognostically and usually respond to antipsychotic medication. An abrupt onset with good premorbid functioning is usually a favourable prognostic sign. A slow insidious onset over a period of 2 or 3 years is more ominous' (Varcarolis 1998, p. 631)

Sadly, there is a high risk of suicide in this group of people, so risk assessment is a key part of any care plan. 'Attempted suicide is a frequent event in the lives of people with schizophrenia, and actual death occurs ... 20 times higher than in the general population' (Lipton and Cancro 1995, cited in Varcarolis 1998, p. 636).

There is a well established belief that stress is a major factor in triggering relapse in people with a schizophrenic predisposition. A stress trigger is believed to be the high level of expressed emotion (HEE) in the families of some people – 'families in which relationships are critical, hostile, dominant, over-involved and with high levels of face-to-face contact' (Brown *et al.* 1972, cited in Thomas *et al.* 1998, p. 229)

Nursing interventions need to be thoughtful, in terms of not reinforcing or colluding with a person's delusional beliefs while at the same time not dismissing their thoughts as having no basis. 'Patients need to helped to develop ways of testing out their delusional beliefs for themselves' (Thomas *et al.* p. 230). The nurse also needs to be prepared for the long-term nature of effective interventions needed. Personal tenacity is very helpful. 'When the nurse is feeling frustrated, it helps to remember that progress often follows an uneven course' (Varcarolis 1998, p. 640).

An experience of nursing a person with schizophrenia

A description of a person with a schizophrenic-type illness may be helpful. You may be able to tell even before you speak to the person that their demeanour is not quite right. There is often something different about their posture, or gait, or both. There is often something about the person that makes them different, even within their usual environment. It can sometimes feel as if there is an invisible sheet of glass between you and them that somehow interferes with or impairs the sort of communication that you would normally expect.

Sufferers may display clusters of symptoms or behaviours and attitudes that make them difficult to approach and engage with, and may cause them, in turn, to be hesitant about approaching us (Gelder *et al.* 1999, Stuart and Laraia 2001, p. 411) They may prefer to position themselves on the perimeters of social groups, although sometimes it might be that they have been positioned there deliberately by society.

Their style of presentation may be just not quite right, or incongruous, in terms of their choice of clothing and way of wearing it. Their eye contact may feel not quite appropriate. There may be other signs that the person does not somehow 'fit' socially, but these can be hard to identify. It's sometimes just a subjective 'feel', in the absence of anything more concrete or objective.

This does not, however, represent all people who suffer with this disorder. Clarke (1999, p. 13) points out that 'Some people with schizophrenia lead reasonable, productive lives'. There is little doubt, though, that sufferers are often socially disabled (Lysaker and Bell 1995, Kane 1999) and experience 'social drift'.

The more experience you have with people who suffer from this dysfunction/illness/disorder, the quicker you seem able to detect it subjectively – i.e. in the absence of little tangible evidence. Of course, thorough objective assessment and time spent with the person can often confirm the initial diagnosis, and hence the nursing treatment strategy, if treatment is needed or desired (sometimes we see it as needed but the patient does not desire it).

The problems can be compounded by the environment, both physically and socially (Suhail 2002, Van Os 2003). The traditional debate follows the themes of whether people suffering from schizophrenia tend to come from poorer social groups or whether they gravitate towards these social settings because of the disabling nature of the illness. This is known in some texts as 'social drift'. Other views are that the person can live at any level of social grouping provided they have consistent and understanding support (Gelder *et al.* 1999, p. 178).

The following case study will give you some idea of how this can look.

PHILIP

Philip Porter is a 35-year-old man originally from Manchester (he says). He has just been admitted to a local acute mental health ward. According to his version of events, his father left the family when Philip was 7 years old. He has some recollection of violence by his father towards his mother. He remembers being woken up at night by 'the fighting and the rows'. He is unwilling to talk any more about his family at this stage.

He reports that he has had a succession of jobs but never manages to settle for longer than a few months as he gets 'picked on' by people at work. This causes him to leave. He is, we note, socially skilled enough to be able to *get* work. The literature on this suggests that, although this type of illness is very disabling in terms of its impact on relationship and job prospects, some sufferers do manage to function relatively well in terms of their ability to stay in stable relationships and employment. Philip says that he has spent long periods of his life regularly going into hospital. Many times he has been admitted when he has been in a period of unemployment. This has always been unwillingly, although he has only been sectioned on a few occasions. He usually feels settled in hospital quite quickly.

He has a younger sister but has lost touch with her. He keeps to himself, stays in bed for long periods and generally isolates himself from both other patients and the nursing staff. He is noted by the nursing staff as being very hard to engage with, giving single-word responses to most attempts to interact with him, with little eye contact and a retiring nature. He seems to be constantly on the retreat from any interaction.

Dialogue with Philip at this stage might look something like this:

Nurse. Hi, Mr Porter, how's it going for you?

This is an open question, the rationale being to provide maximum opportunity for Philip to 'engage'. Also, it is worth considering whether you use the familiar first name or stay more formal. In this instance our approach is more tentative and respectful. The use of a first name could be felt as over-familiar and even intrusive, so unless you are sure of yourself use the formal approach first. The permission to use first names, if and when it comes, is a helpful way of keeping some power with the patient (empowering) in a situation where they may feel almost powerless.

Philip. OK (*breaks off eye contact*).
Nurse. Good, see you later.

The rationale here is to indicate to Philip that the relationship has some sense of, or potential for, continuity. This must be followed up, as trust is a major issue here.

Here the nurse is still trying to do several things in what looks to the casual observer like a very superficial interaction:

- Start to establish some kind of relaxed conversational 'habit' or routine between them. This is laying the foundations of a 'rapport'. The routine and thus relatively unthreatening nature of this can help Philip to start to feel a little safer in what, for him, can be an unsettling or even frightening environment at first, even if he is relatively used to the role of 'patient' and what that entails. Many people who suffer with schizophrenia feel frightened and on edge (Stuart and Laraia 2001, p.415).

- Even if it takes the nurse days or weeks to get further than this, at least Philip is being regularly assessed and monitored.

- The nurse is demonstrating some level of care and concern and just ordinary friendliness. People with Philip's background or history may not be used to this because the illness is so socially isolating (Hochberger 1992). It takes a level of skill and sensitivity to not overdo this on the part of the nurse. It must not be perceived as a pressure by the patient, otherwise it could be more destructive than constructive. Perhaps 'little and often' could be a useful rule of thumb. There is little point in pushing at this stage as there is a strong likelihood that you will alienate Philip. That is a role he is used to occupying anyway.

Nurse. Hi, Mr Porter – is that what you like to be called? Have you seen today's paper/How about a cup of tea?/Do you want to watch TV for a bit?

The rationale here is to demonstrate the continuity mentioned above, to further assess and to further demonstrate that you care/are bothered/are OK/are approachable.

Philip. No I'm not bothered,
Nurse. OK, Philip, I'll try you again in a bit.

The rationale here is again to demonstrate that there is some sort of commitment from you (and perhaps later on from other members of the nursing staff). Note that the nurse is trying to use an approach that is tentative, non-intrusive and yet gently persistent.

Philip's prognosis (the potential course of the illness) is difficult to predict.

Traditional thinking suggests a high chance of chronic disablement with regular stress-induced relapses. Current thinking suggests that if this unique cluster of relapse symptoms ('relapse signature' – Meadows 2003) can be detected at an early stage the relapse can perhaps be 'nipped in the bud' by early intervention or can be proactively nursed to reduce the severity of the relapse (Newell and Gournay 2000, p. 155).

Depending on the nature of Philip's illness the next stage of the interventions could be something like this:

Nurse. Morning Philip. How's it going for you today?
Philip. Not so bad. I was a bit shaky last night, the voices really started on me again.
Nurse. What happened?

This one could be seen as a breakthrough, in terms of you getting something back. He is starting to let you help, or at least checking your commitment to try. An alternative response, though, could be more like this:

Nurse. Morning Philip. How's it going for you today?
Philip. What's it got to fucking do with you lot? Leave me alone.
Nurse. OK. See you later. (*It is important to say this in a neutral but friendly way*)

This second response hints at the existence of a person suffering with 'positive symptoms' of the illness (Charlton 2000) that have still to react to medication. If this is so, then the nurses still interact with a calm, consistent, stable, predictable, non-confrontational approach. If Philip experiences this approach as a reaction to his aggression and lack of trust, the chances of him acquiescing are greatly increased.

The next stage is the response to the deluded patient. There are several key principles to remember here. The main one is, don't argue with the person who is experiencing delusional thought because you are likely to increase their level of distress and agitation. For example, a person who is experiencing the delusional idea that they are HIV-positive can be shown the results of their blood test indicating a negative result. They may then denounce this as a fake because it's someone else's result, or suggest that there is a plot to deceive them. The nursing response, therefore, can only usefully be neutral, but with a longer-term intention to at least not reinforce the delusion. The patient will be using much energy to do that themselves. For example Philip, during a bad patch, says:

You're trying to paralyse me with these drugs. You'll never get me to take them again.

The immediate implications of this are serious. A possible consequence of this thinking by Philip might be for him to be sectioned under the Mental Health Act (1983) and given a course of medication anyway. This could happen if he continually refused to accept antipsychotics and his delusional state gave cause for concern about his safety or that of others. The Mental Health Act is used often to arrange assessment and/or treatment of people who are otherwise unwilling to do this voluntarily. Meanwhile, anything resembling a therapeutic relationship is at risk as the staff head towards the classic paradox in mental health nursing – that of the custodial role overlying the caring role (Coombs 1996). Some of the possible responses to Philip's statement might be:

What makes you say that Philip? (Asking for more information – Catalytic)
You sound really angry, Philip. (Responding to the emotion, trying to be empathic)
Why would we want to paralyse you, Philip? (Seeing if a Socratic approach might work)
What do you mean, Philip? (Trying to clarify)

Some of the aims behind these approaches are to keep dialogue going, demonstrate concern and show interest. Note that in every example his name is used and the nature of the interaction is open and encourages a further exchange.

There is of course a risk with this style of interaction. The risk is that we are now tightly focused on one of Philip's most powerful ideas. This may be a central part of his world at the moment. The risk is that these beliefs might become even more entrenched. Outweighing this risk are the probable benefits of loosening the ties that bind him to such ideas and trying to create some room to manoeuvre for him and his carers. If you can keep the dialogue going you are increasing the chances of sustaining the therapeutic relationship, which will probably be under threat at this stage.

Summary of skills used ▶

- Open questions are used to help develop dialogue as much as possible
- A tentative approach is maintained, especially in the early stages of the relationship
- The relationship is one of respect and encourages empowerment
- A major aim is the development of a friendly trusting rapport
- The carers try to be approachable and ordinary
- They work collaboratively
- They are gently persistent and consistent
- The interventions go at a pace that the patient is capable of.

4.2 PEOPLE WHO ARE ABNORMALLY OVERACTIVE

Introduction

People who are abnormally overactive may also be known as manic, hypomanic or bipolar.

Some of the signs of this disorder are: 'marked impairment in judgement, often leading to serious legal, social, occupational, or interpersonal consequences ... constant physical activity, pressured speech, and racing thought patterns, irritability may be the predominant mood disturbance, may begin suddenly and last a few days to months, grandiose or persecutory delusions' (Varcarolis 1998, pp. 596–597). There are important issues here with safety of the person, and others, because of their unpredictable behaviour. There is risk also of the patient becoming physically ill through dehydration or malnutrition. There are particular problems with younger people. 'Hypomania, when it presents in teenagers, is often dramatic, difficult to treat and very challenging to work with' (Thomas *et al.* 1998, p. 342).

Nursing interventions are essentially directed towards the safety and physical health of the person together with a focus on keeping them within a calming environment. Using distracting tactics is helpful, when appropriate, together with a 'firm and neutral approach' (Varcarolis 1998, p. 604). A collaborative and consistent approach is needed as in this mental state patients can be liable to 'taunt the staff by pointing out faults or oversights, drawing negative attention to one or more staff, divide staff as a ploy to keep the environment unsettled' (Varcarolis 1998, p. 604).

An experience of nursing someone with hypomania

This can often feel like a balancing act – you are trying to keep the relationship safe (superficial as it may be) but there seems to be the ever-present danger that it will tip towards instability. People who are in a hypomanic or manic state tend to be on high alert and have an ability to concentrate on every detail of everything you say to them. Some care and thoughtfulness is therefore needed to navigate through any conversation you become involved in. This is not to suggest that the nurse needs to acquiesce to everything that the person is saying in an attempt to 'humour' him/her. Any attempt to do this is likely to backfire as it is surprising how sensitive people with this condition are to being patronised.

It might be useful to try to see things from the sufferer's viewpoint, although, paradoxically, sufferers often see themselves as anything but suffering. Their liberal philosophy of life can suddenly change to an over-reactive style of dealing with situations around them. This modifying of personality can also, unfortunately, sometimes tip into aggressive interactions, which makes people with this disorder very tiring to be around and very tiring to nurse proactively and thoughtfully. Add to this the reactions of other people (patients and sometimes even staff) to an irritable or inappropriately humorous person, and the nurse can find him/herself in the role of peacemaker within a volatile community.

ERIC

Eric is a 40-year-old unemployed man with a long history of admissions to the mental health unit. He has a very supportive partner who recognises that Eric often reacts to stressful situations by becoming unwell. She finds him very difficult to manage, however, as he becomes more and more verbally aggressive towards her, and females in general. Eric has been on the ward for three days and is very unpredictable in his moods. The atmosphere on the ward is tense:

Eric. Are you the matron of this dump? How come all your nurses sit around drinking tea and smoking? Shouldn't they be helping us lot get better? I'm going to see my MP about this place – it's crap.
Nurse. Some of the nurses have a cup of tea or a cigarette as it's a good opportunity to sit with people on the ward and get to know them a bit better. We do that with you a lot, don't we?
Eric. What do you mean get to know them? Is that so the nurses can have it off with them? You're all the same, sex mad.

> **Nurse.** Sitting with people is the best way we know to just listen to their problems. That's how we try to help.
> **Eric.** Typical. An answer for everything.

You will see that there is no comfortable resolution to this conversation. Often the nurse has a sense that whatever they say they will not 'win around' the person, who seems hell bent on picking away at every perceived fault in whatever system they are a part of at the moment (a hospital ward, day hospital, their own home). Perhaps a helpful aim could be towards a therapeutic relationship, which, in part, could entail the nurse behaving in a predictably consistent 'firm but fair way'. This would also, of course, reflect the aims of the individual patient's plan of care.

This is a highly skilled type of nursing given the needs of other patients/clients and the usual routines and demands that are part of any institutional care setting. If the patient's perception is that s/he will be listened to in a way that is stable, reasonable, consistent, adult and non-patronising, then the chances are that, if and when the medication starts to temper the high activity levels, the re-socialising process can be much more rapid – re-establishing the person's usual communication habits, which have helped them manage prior to the onset of the overactive period.

> **Eric.** Why does everybody in this fucking place keep moaning at me? I was just trying to tidy everybody's locker. This place is like a tip.
> **Nurse.** It's good of you to try to help. We usually let people deal with their own lockers. I'm nipping out to get a newspaper soon. Do you fancy having a change of scene?
> **Eric.** Anything to get away from this miserable lot.
> **Nurse.** Good. Are you going to sort out your shoes and a coat? It's getting cold out now.
> **Eric.** OK. With you in a minute.

Here the aim of the nurse is to gradually bring down Eric's agitated mood. Eric's irritation with other people on the ward is diverted into something constructive. The idea of removing him from this environment to somewhere else – perhaps less stimulating – will be congruent with, and support, the approach of using medication that will also tend towards mellowing his volatility.

Summary of skills used ▷

- Nursing interventions are firm and neutral
- A consistent approach is used
- The interventions are carried out thoughtfully in terms of looking after the person's safety and physical health
- The intention is likely to be predominantly informative and prescriptive
- Non-verbal communication (eye contact, proxemics) is used in a considered way, as there may be heightened sensitivity to these
- A non-stimulating environment is sought out for the patient wherever possible

4.3 PEOPLE WHO ARE WITHDRAWN/LOW IN MOOD/DEPRESSED/DYSTHYMIC

Introduction

Some texts have described this condition as the 'common cold' of psychiatry. At its worst the sufferer is overcome with feelings and thoughts of hopelessness: 'profound, persistent and all pervasive, a sadness, helplessness ... self-esteem is low' (Thomas *et al.* 1998, p. 238). Varcarolis (1998, p. 559) points out that: 'grooming, dress, and personal hygiene are markedly neglected'.

There are no quick fixes here. The experience of nursing someone who is depressed, which follows, is based in a mental health ward setting. It is important to point out that most people who suffer from depression are treated in a community setting (Thomas *et al.* 1998). Unfortunately, although some depression seems to be treatable, most people who suffer with depression experience multiple episodes (Varcarolis 1998).

Some depression seems to be reactive, i.e. it occurs in response to events in the person's life. Other people find it difficult to pinpoint or attribute any specific reason for it. 'Many people state that they have no reason to be depressed, and they cannot identify any problems or environmental stressors in their lives' (Varcarolis 1998, p. 553).

An experience of nursing someone who is depressed

Nursing interventions are likely to focus around the safety of the patient. Suicide risk will be assessed and monitored. If the person is severely retarded their basic needs (hydration, nutrition, hygiene) will be looked after. Medication compliance will be monitored. Even though some people respond well to contemporary anti depressants, some do not. A cognitive approach can sometimes be the most effective choice of the 'talking' interventions, together with Rogerian core attributes (see also section 2.11). Also, as Varcarolis (1998, p. 564) notes: 'Just sitting with a patient in silence may seem like a waste of time to the nurse ... it is important to be aware that this time spent together can be meaningful to the depressed person'.

Ordinary approaches such as regular offers of tea/drinks, to look at a paper or the TV may be rejected or ignored. Gentle persistence may pay off in terms of the person starting to show the first sign of a willingness to communicate. This may only be slightly longer eye contact at first, rather than words.

SALLY

Sally was admitted to an acute unit a couple of days ago.

Nurse. Morning, Sally. Get any sleep?
Sally. Not really.
Nurse. Try not to worry too much about that. You'll catch up when you're ready. Even a couple of hours is better than nothing. It's understandable that your sleep is disturbed, given what's happened, and that you're in a strange environment. How about some breakfast?
Sally. I'll give it a miss. I don't usually bother at home.
Nurse. I'll bring you a cup of tea in a while. See how you go.

One of the nurse's aims over the short term is to be supportive, reassuring and informative while observing and monitoring. Over the next few hours a longer-term aim is to keep re-establishing contact with Sally. There are several benefits to this in terms of the person's care:

- The person's mood (affect) can be monitored
- The relationship can be nurtured towards a therapeutic one
- Opportunities are created for the person to talk
- The person may feel valued and noticed – low self-esteem is often connected closely with depressive tendencies (McGovern and Whitcher 1994).

> **Nurse.** Hi, Sally. How about going for a walk with me for 20 minutes?
> **Sally.** No I'm all right.
> **Nurse.** There's a patients' meeting in about an hour. You'd be very welcome. You don't have to say anything.
> **Sally.** No, I'm OK, thanks. Meetings aren't my cup of tea.
> **Nurse.** Some other time perhaps. They are once a week in the day room. If you want anything from the shop, let me know and we could walk down together. You must be sick of looking at these walls.
> **Sally.** Yes, but I'd rather be here than in that flat.
> **Nurse.** What was so bad about the flat?
> **Sally.** It was starting to feel like a prison?
> **Nurse.** How do you mean – a prison?

Here the nurse has continued the strategy of ordinariness in the conversational themes at the start of this conversation. The intention is to re-socialise, re-engage Sally into something diverting. There is further investment in a relationship that may eventually become therapeutic for Sally.

The comment by the nurse: 'You must be sick of looking at these walls' has a deliberate aim. It is not a casual remark. It has an empathic aim to it. Another intention is to assess and at the same time provide more opportunity for Sally to start talking about her experience 'here and now' as a patient, and her experiences in the past. The nurse's tentative use of open questions gently encourages Sally to start exploring her experiences. The insights this could give the nurse may be very useful in terms of additional data to help the care team help Sally.

It is essential that the nurse makes it clear to Sally, before the conversation is developed any further, that parts of the conversation may be relayed back to the care team in an effort to help her. Sally's consent for this must be obtained now, not at a later stage.

> **Sally.** Every night when I got back from work, it felt like the walls were closing in. It seemed as if the phone never rang any more. People didn't care about me. I was in solitary confinement ... well, that's how it felt.
> **Nurse.** Sounds like it was a horrible time for you. How did you deal with that feeling?
> **Sally.** Sometimes I drank a bit. Sometimes I just went to bed early. Then I couldn't sleep. I just lay there.
> **Nurse.** How long did that go on for?
> **Sally.** Right up to when I decided to end it.

The nurse is letting the conversation develop. The bulk of the talking is being done by Sally. Any intervention by the nurse at this stage is aimed towards consolidating the start of the therapeutic relationship and encouraging Sally to deepen her disclosure. This is to gain more insight and understanding into Sally's condition, rather than for intrusive reasons. The nurse almost holds back at this stage. She is tentative and sensitive. She tries not to cause Sally to suddenly feel under pressure or a sense of being cajoled into disclosure.

The approach demonstrated above could be typical of a constructive strategy to helping people with depression in that it contains several important characteristics:

- A therapeutic relationship is constantly being aimed for
- Diversion is used thoughtfully
- Information about the subjective experience of the person is always being sought (This is essential in terms of assessing risk of self harm/suicide)
- An empathic approach is attempted (Sometimes this is effective, sometimes not. It is always worth the effort)
- An intrusive or pushy approach is avoided
- The person's own imagery is used (i.e. prison).

The likelihood is that Sally will have been prescribed a course of antidepressants. The nursing interventions described above, together with appropriate medication, are likely to help Sally start on the way back to recovery. The role of other more structured approaches, such as cognitive behavioural therapy, psychotherapy or a problem-solving approach may become apparent as the care team finds out more about Sally's needs.

Summary of skills used ▶

- Gentle persistence
- Reassuring
- Open questions
- Ordinariness
- Diverting when appropriate
- Empathic approach
- Acceptance
- Tentativeness
- Use of imagery

4.4 People who have abnormally difficult personalities

Introduction

People who are labelled with this diagnosis (which may also be called personality disorder, sociopath, psychopath, PD) carry with them a stigma even within professional circles. Some professionals see them as especially challenging and others see them as untreatable: 'Many mental health professionals approach this client group with a mixture of reluctance and apprehension' (Jones 2002, p. 6). Certainly, it is widely acknowledged that any signs that treatment has been effective will be a long time in coming: 'PD has a generally poor outcome ... [there is] ... widespread therapeutic pessimism' (Jones 2002, p. 6). This of course has cost implications. Aronson (1989, cited in McLeod 1998, p. 46) says that 'The intensity and challenge of this kind of therapeutic work, and the generally moderate success rates associated with it, mean that practitioners are often cautious about taking on borderline [personality disorder] clients'.

It appears that men are more likely to be given this diagnostic label than women (Thomas *et al.* 1998). People with this disorder are difficult to live with and difficult to nurse. It is not clear sometimes if the person has much insight:

> *People with PDs are not always in extreme distress or even emotional discomfort. Often, it is the people who live or work with these individuals who are the most distressed. Manipulation and power struggles are thus the norm in all relationships of a person with PD. Fear of closeness results, and a precarious dance ensues.*
>
> Varcarolis 1998, p. 508

Varcarolis also lists (1998, p. 508) four characteristics that she states are present in 'all of the PDs':

- Inflexible and maladaptive responses to stress
- Disability in working and loving
- Ability to evoke interpersonal conflict
- Capacity to have an intense effect on others (this process is often unconscious and generally produces undesirable results).

There are great difficulties in nursing this group of individuals, given their propensity to cause conflict. Varcarolis (1998, p. 523) suggests: 'exhibit respect and patience, make a genuine attempt to understand the client's experience'. This is a considerable challenge when set against 'these clients tell the nurse that the nurse is inadequate, incompetent, and they are abusive of authority, substantial conflict can ensue in the workplace' (Varcarolis 1998, p. 523).

An experience of nursing someone who has a personality disorder

In many ways patients with this diagnosis are the most challenging group of people to nurse, especially for the beginner. The usual positive human qualities of trust, consistency, reliability and openness seem to disappear, or are well hidden. Try to start with an open mind. You may not even know, at first, like the rest of the care team, that you are talking to a person with a disordered personality. If the person has no previous history in mental health services this set of characteristics may only become gradually apparent over time and with good communication throughout the team.

AMY

Tuesday morning:

> **Nurse.** How's it going today, Amy?
> **Amy.** Not too bad, I suppose. Did you hear about John? He cut himself in the toilet last night again. How did he get those scissors? Will that nurse get

into trouble? He ought to – not doing his job properly. I feel really sorry for that John, he's really screwed up, isn't he? You ought to be his named nurse, he'd be much better off, wouldn't he?

Nurse. Mmmm, who knows? What have you got planned for the rest of today, Amy?

The nurse's intention here is to sustain the rapport with Amy that she already has without getting involved in the tangle of potential traps presented in these few sentences. As you will see from the conversation the day after (below), the quality of this rapport varies greatly from day to day, and even from hour to hour. This is a significant indicator in terms of assessing the type of relationship you have with patients. Some of the characteristics that Amy demonstrates above are:

- Not wishing to engage with the offered intervention
- Getting enmeshed in other patients' problems, and sometimes even becoming part of their problems
- Separating staff members into 'good' and 'bad'
- Tempting/encouraging staff to breach confidentiality and behave in unprofessional ways (some beginner nurses are vulnerable to this)
- Manipulating people in a sometimes naïve/childlike way and sometimes in a very sophisticated way.

Wednesday morning:

Nurse. How's it going today, Amy?

Amy. What do you care? You're all the same – worse than the fucking police, you lot.

Nurse. You seem very different from yesterday when we spoke. What's happened to you?

The nurse's intention here is to attempt to re-engage Amy by not reacting to her abusive remarks while at the same time demonstrating the same level of interest, respect and concern given to all patients. The chances of this are remote. A key approach to personalities like Amy's is a consistent, persistent, adult (Berne 1975) approach over a long period of time.

Notice also that the nurse is now not 'special' any more, and is 'one of them'. This is one of the most difficult things for the beginner nurse to manage. Sometimes remarks are made to you that feel very hurtful in a personal way. This can happen with any patient/client. The experience of being a patient/client can be very frustrating and sometimes this causes feelings of great hostility towards the 'staff'. If the 'staff' at the moment are represented by you, it is possible that you will be the target of a torrent of abuse. The likelihood of this happening is probably greatly increased when the person who is becoming frustrated has a disordered personality. Their ability to be reasonable and empathic are greatly diminished.

Amy. Martin told me that I'd be able to go out this morning. He's not on duty and that nurse in the office said I couldn't go. Martin's the only one who understands me in this hospital. I wish he was my nurse. All the patients say this is the worst ward in the whole hospital. The staff are crap.

Nurse. You still haven't told me what happened to you since yesterday.

Amy. My bloody stepdad rang me. He wound me up again. Are you happy now?

Here the nurse has not become drawn into the relative merits of who are the best members of staff and which is the worst ward. The negative feelings that are aimed at the nurse are taken on board but not openly responded to. They may in truth be upsetting, but it is important to try to remember that a way of managing this type of situation is not to be drawn into personal conflict. What the nurse is trying to do is to help Amy reveal what has triggered off this latest burst of negative energy that she is targeting at the staff.

There are several important steps the nurse should take now to ensure that the interaction and the nurse's deliberate and thoughtful intervention are used to maximum therapeutic effect:

- The opportunity could be taken to encourage Amy to express her feelings about her stepfather, if appropriate. A decision needs to be made on the spot. Whether this can be contained, or if it is likely to escalate out of control, needs to be considered. Very negative repercussions such as restraint could be an extreme consequence. In this type of situation, if you have any doubt, a better course of action is to give Amy the opportunity to deal with it in her own way under the monitoring eye of the staff. After all, this is what she has to do when she is not in a care setting.
- The more experienced staff on the team need to be told. They may wish to use the opportunity to approach Amy differently.
- The incident should be logged in Amy's care notes. It may not be clear at this point how significant the contact with Amy's stepfather is.
- It would be important to explore this with Amy at some future appropriate time. This in itself would be considered carefully, as it might possibly cause Amy to become agitated again.
- Martin will be asked whether he did sanction or suggest that Amy could go home. Not so that punitive action could be taken, but to ascertain whether or not staff are acting independently from each other or whether Amy is deliberately splitting staff away from the main group.

The interaction continues:

Nurse. What is it about your step-dad that makes you so angry? Every time he rings you get like this. It seems to really get to you.
Amy. Yes it's driving me mad. I could kill him. Why doesn't he leave me alone?
Nurse. So what's going on?
Amy. I want to talk to Martin. He'll help. I can't talk to you.

Here the nurse has decided that she knows Amy well enough to continue the strategy of asking open questions. She is trying to understand Amy's situation in more depth. She tries to empathise but the attempt seems to be wasted. It is still worth an attempt, though. This is what helps to make the effective mental health nurse – the ability to be gently persistent, creative and optimistic. One day it might work, and that could represent a small breakthrough in a long process with Amy. Once again, at the end of this interaction Amy turns on the nurse and resumes the strategy of splitting the staff into good (Mark) and bad (the nurse). This is to be expected. It is what she knows.

Discussion point

Are people who have a disordered personality suffering from a mental illness? If so, in what way? Haven't we all got disordered personalities to some extent? Read through the Personality Clusters in the DSM-IV (American Psychiatric Association 1994) and see how many times you spot your own personal characteristics.

Summary of skills used ▶

- Trying to create a rapport – despite the inherent difficulties
- Being consistent and persistent
- Maintaining a respectful attitude
- Attempting to be empathic
- Being thoughtful with intentions
- Working in a collaborative way
- Making use of your supervision

4.5 PEOPLE WHO HAVE ORGANIC MENTAL ILLNESS

Introduction

Organic mental illnesses include dementia, Alzheimer's disease, Korsakoff's disease, Pick's disease, multi-infarct disease, Creutzfeldt–Jakob disease, Lewy body disease and Parkinson's disease (see also Thomas *et al.* 1998).

Alzheimer's disease probably accounts for up to 70% of all cases of dementia (Varcarolis 1998, p. 714). Some of the characteristics of Alzheimer's dementia are described thus by Varcarolis (1998, p. 691–693): 'Deterioration may be subtle and insidious, it attacks indiscriminately, disorganisation of personality [will] occur, [it is] marked by progressive deterioration in intellectual functioning, memory, and ability to solve problems and learn new skills'. There are of course consequences for the relatives and significant others, who may experience feelings of loss for the person they knew. 'The effects of losing a family member to dementia can be devastating' (Varcarolis 1998, p. 701).

The nursing interventions are focused on safety, physical needs and an understanding of the process of the disease, combined with an acceptance of the struggles of the person who suffers with it. 'The nurse's attitude of unconditional positive regard is the single most effective tool in caring for demented clients' (Varcarolis 1998, p. 701).

An experience of nursing someone with an organic mental illness

EDNA

The starting point for the skills needed to effectively communicate with this group of people is the realisation that often (but not always) your normal interventions may be responded to in strange ways. For example:

> **Nurse.** Hi, Edna. Are you ready for some lunch?
> **Edna.** Where's Bill? I need to get his tea ready. He'll be home soon. I need to get on. (*Bill, her husband, died some years ago*)

There are several ways to respond to Edna in this situation. The most caring, sensitive and humane way to handle it is often to attempt to reflect the feeling or emotion behind Edna's words. It is likely that in this instance they reflect her desire to get things done for when her husband returns. Maybe this was a regular occurrence in their earlier life together. Perhaps she would be preparing a meal for his return from work. The feeling behind her words might be a need to get the job done properly and to keep to a well-established routine. She may also be feeling perhaps a little frustration at this person (the nurse) who is getting in the way of, or interfering with, the process.

> **Nurse.** It must be irritating for you that I'm getting in the way, Edna. How about we get you something to eat and drink, then you can get on with the rest of the day? Let's make sure you're OK first.

The nurse's intention here is:

- To respond directly and genuinely to Edna's frustration
- To re-focus on the immediate nursing needs of Edna, i.e. to provide her with food and drink
- Not to reinforce Edna's need to look after her husband
- To re-focus the whole interaction back on to Edna
- Not to become involved in the reality that Edna's husband has been dead for several years.

The principle above of trying to respond to the feeling in the words of the patient uses a technique called *validation therapy* (Norman and Redfern 1997). Another approach that should be given consideration by the effective nurse is *reality orientation* (Norman and Redfern 1997). As you would imagine, this is the technique of using the reality of the patient's situation to help them. Again, this has to be used with care and thoughtfulness. As carers we must constantly ask the question: What is the benefit *to the patient* of reinforcing the reality of their situation? Would you respond to Edna, for example, by saying:

> Bill died a long time ago, Edna. Let's concentrate on getting you some tea.

Some carers might use this approach, but what does it achieve in terms of the comfort of the patient?

Sometimes a combination of the validation approach and the reality approach can seem to work well for the patient, in terms of the helpfulness of the intervention for the patient's comfort:

> **Nurse.** Edna, it's nearly time for your evening meal. Would you like to get ready?
> **Edna.** Ooh, you are good in this hotel. Could I have the bill soon? I'm not sure if I've got enough money on me.
> **Nurse.** Don't worry Edna you don't need to pay any bills here. That's all taken care of. Now, which pair of shoes would you like to wear this evening, Edna?

All the above techniques can be used by the beginner nurse. Your effectiveness will fluctuate. Be persistent and as consistent as you are able. Try to consider what you are saying. These thoughtful interventions, together with an increase in the use of more physical skills such as touch, when appropriate, might compensate for deficits in the elderly person's repertoire of senses and skills. They can make a significant impact on the quality of their life as a person in your care.

> **Edna.** I don't know which pair. Bill likes the blue ones best. Let's get them. That'll please him.
> **Nurse.** Good choice. You look nice in those. Shall we go through to the dining room now?
> **Edna.** Yes please, I'm a bit peckish now. Will Bill be able to find us? Does he know I'm in this hotel?
> **Nurse.** You'll be fine. Come on, follow me. Take it steady. (*Guides Edna gently by the arm, as she is a little wobbly*)

Summary of skills used ▷

- Gentle persistence
- Consistency
- Touch
- Eye contact
- Appropriate use of reality and validation techniques
- Acceptance
- Empathic person-centred approach

4.6 ABNORMAL SELF-DESTRUCTIVE BEHAVIOURS

Introduction

Such behaviours might include substance abuse, eating disorders and self-harm.

Certain characteristics seem to be common among people who are self-destructive in different ways.

- 'There is always the awareness of the tension between treatment and social control' (drugs and alcohol; Thomas *et al.* 1998, p. 306)
- 'High levels of therapist frustration, treatment resistance and non-compliance are reported by therapists' (eating disorders; Burkett and Schramm 1995, cited in Thomas *et al.* 1998, p. 314)
- 'A sense of release is experienced' (self-harm; Bywaters and, Rolfe 2002, p. 21; see also Johnstone 2000)
- 'May be anxious about recovering because to do so they must give up the [abusive behaviour] they think they need to survive (drug abuse; Varcarolis 1998, p. 767)
- 'Manipulative behaviours seen in these clients may lead nurses to feel angry and exploited (drug abuse; Varcarolis 1998, p. 771)
- 'Nurses should ask questions in a matter-of-fact non-judgemental way' (drug abuse; Varcarolis 1998, p. 754)
- 'Central to participants' positive accounts were attitudes: tolerance, trying to

understand and treating them like a person and with respect' (self-harm, Bywaters and Rolfe 2002, p. 22)

- 'Women who self harm have described their greatest needs as being for someone to listen, accept, respect and help them to explore their underlying problems and release their pain and anger in different ways' (Johnstone 2000, p. 115).

Nursing people who exhibit self-destructive behaviours is sometimes carried out in specialist mental health settings. However. the mental health student is very likely to encounter people with some of these problems in the acute setting. The interventions described in this section and Section 5.9 are intended to help the beginner in the early stages of work with this group.

An experience of nursing someone who displays self-destructive behaviours

This is another area of disorder that mental health nurses will have to address, as self-harm is an increasing problem (Hawton 2001, Gelder *et al.* 1999, Jacobson and Jacobson 1996, Newell and Gournay 2000), and this is another group of people you will inevitably encounter during your training. It is likely that the number of people affected by such disorders (not just the immediate sufferers but relatives and friends as well) will increase over the next few years as neither the misuse of non-prescription drugs (Department of Health 2003) nor the obsession with image (Simpson 2002) show any sign of abating:

JAYNE

Jayne is a 20-year-old student. She has had several brief admissions to the local acute ward. Her parents are very worried and upset. They wonder: 'What have we done wrong? Her sister's OK.' Jayne is under threat of being terminated from her course because of high sickness rate and unexplained absences. She appears unconcerned about this.

Nurse. Jayne what have you done to your arm?
Jayne. I've cut it again.
Nurse. Let's have a look at it. What triggered it off this time? (*This is said in a calm way, with no judgement implied*)
Jayne. I just needed to do it. It feels better now.
Nurse. Come into the clinic and we'll clean it up. It would help if you could find one of us to talk to when you feel like doing this. I know you don't always want to. Maybe we could help you find another way to deal with this rather than cutting. (*Again said in a non-judgemental way*)
Jayne. It feels so good though, like a relief.

This illustrates a dilemma concerning treatment of people who self-harm frequently. The act of self-harm is sometimes a response to the psychological pain experienced and in fact a release of tension is commonly experienced: 'a sense of release, calm, just a stillness' (Bywaters and Rolfe 2002, p. 21). This makes it very difficult for members of the care team to offer a more attractive alternative. The ritual of self-harming is the response that the person knows is usually reliable. The aim of the thoughtful nurse as always, can be 'multilayered' (Bywaters and Rolfe 2002).

- The act of self-harm must be accepted (but not encouraged)
- No judgement should be communicated, neither disapproval or approval
- Alternative responses should be indicated
- Solutions should not be suggested
- Practical nursing care should be offered
- The person should not be rejected in any way – 'Central to participants' positive accounts were attitudes: tolerance, trying to understand and treating them like a person and with respect' (Bywaters and Rolfe 2002, p. 22).

Nurse. How would it be, if when you experience these feelings, you try to divert yourself away from cutting by talking to one of us? There's always someone here to sit with you. You may find that over time it could be helpful for you.

Jayne. I'd rather just cut. It always helps. You lot are too busy anyway.

Nurse. I'll talk to your key worker and we'll try to arrange it so that if you feel bad then there will be someone for you. Ben would agree with that, wouldn't he? How about talking it over with him as well? (*Ben is Jayne's partner*)

The nurse is still being quietly persistent in trying to persuade Jayne to deal with her self-harm habit in a more constructive way. She aims to assure Jayne of a consistent approach from her colleagues in the care team. She thinks maybe that a supportive partner might also be able to exert gentle pressure on her to attempt to change her behaviour.

Jayne. He probably would. I don't want to get him involved in this any more, though. I've put him through enough already.

Nurse. Well, think about it, will you?

Summary of skills used ▶

- Accepting of the person but not the behaviour
- Consistent
- Constructive
- Communicative to other care team members
- Calm, persistent, problem-solving approach (Newell and Gournay 2000)

5 ILLUSTRATIVE STORIES

These stories bring the practical skills in Chapters 1–3 together with their application to disorders illustrated in Chapter 4. They are then set into a wider context than in Chapter 4. The rationale for this is that, when people become mentally ill, a sequence of unique events (for that person) is initiated. For example, at the start of a depressive episode a person may start to feel 'odd' – not themselves – out of sorts. Is it that they are just 'run down'? Is it the start of 'flu or some other physical illness? Is it stress, work problems, relationship problems, financial difficulties, spiritual uncertainty, mid-life crisis, destructive peer-group pressure (drugs, slimming), even a combination of several of these? The stories try to take account of the impact of these precursors to connecting with mental health services, not only on the patient or client but on their relatives and significant others.

Many of us experience some of these precursors at some points in our lives. Newbigging (2002) suggests that up to 40% of people consulting their GP have a mental health problem. Three out of four of us manage or cope but one in four will need psychiatric intervention; some of those will go on to develop psychiatric illness that becomes an established part of their life, and some of those will die as a result of this illness. Armson (2003, p. 14) states that, statistically, 'the average primary care group with a population of 100 000 can expect 10 suicides a year'.

The feature common to all those who go on to experience diagnosable mental illness is that they travel along a pathway or 'journey to recovery' (Department of Health 2002b). This unique route can sometimes be positively influenced by skilled and thoughtful interventions from professional carers. The stories in this chapter indicate how the skills, techniques and ideas described earlier, once they are understood, can be used to help student carers, sufferers and their significant others. They are not intended to be prescriptive, but suggest how interventions could be.

5.1 MENTAL HEALTH PROBLEMS IN OUR SOCIETY – SETTING THE SCENE

There is no clear distinction between mental health and mental disorder. We all exist on a continuum of emotional 'ups and downs' and imperfect perceptual interpretations of our environment. Our lives are an uncertain mixture of comedy and tragedy and, as any fictional drama demonstrates, our relationships with others are characterised as much by conflict and the need to reduce tension as by compatibility and harmony. We all struggle at times to maintain emotional and social competence.

Some psychologists suggest that 'good' mental health is demonstrated by such attributes as:

- Efficient perception of reality
- An ability to exercise voluntary control over behaviour
- Self-esteem and acceptance

- An ability to form affectionate relationships that are mutually supportive
- An ability to channel behaviour into productive activity (Atkinson *et al.* 1996).

Discussion point

Identify additional attributes, including those that contribute to 'happiness'. What makes unhappiness or periods of severe emotional distress bearable or endurable?

Periods of distress in life are unavoidable, and some people seem to experience more than their fair share. There is no distinct cut-off point at which emotional disturbance, or eccentricity, or other differences, might be regarded as significantly 'abnormal'. Such judgements can often only be made by consideration of individual circumstances, and may still be controversial.

Nevertheless, psychiatrists, psychologists and other human scientists recognise a number of distinct conditions or syndromes that occur with sufficient regularity and predictability to be formally classified as 'illnesses' or 'disorders'.

There are two main classification systems of mental disorder that are used to guide formal diagnosis by appropriate professionals. One is the World Health Organization's International Classification of Diseases, which is now into its 10th edition (ICD-10). The other is the American Psychiatric Association's Diagnostic and Statistical Manual of Diseases, which is now into its fourth edition (DSM-IV; American Psychiatric Association 1994). There are some variations between these, which, together with the constant revisions, have served to strengthen the views of the critics of psychiatry, who regard diagnostic labels as stigmatising and lacking scientific validity. Some people question whether it is helpful to regard 'mental illness' as illness, since this implies physical causes and medical treatments.

Mental illness is estimated to affect up to one in four adults at some stage of their lives. Mental illness serious enough to need professional assistance is suffered by one in 10 people (Health of the Nation 1992)

Family doctors in Britain make 4,000,000 diagnoses a year of emotional or psychological disorder (according to the Audit Commission). Of these, 1,000,000 a year are referred to specialist mental health services. There are 200,000 admissions to in-patient services, of which about 10% are admitted compulsorily. This percentage is steadily increasing. People are admitted in this way for being a danger to themselves or others (Gelder *et al.* 1999). The majority of these people are mainly a danger to themselves. Over 55,000 people commit suicide each year – more than the number who die in road traffic accidents (Department of Health 1992). This figure has been rising steadily for some years despite repeated government initiatives to reduce the incidence. By contrast, the number of homicides committed annually by people with a serious mental disorder has been static for some decades (Laurance 2003).

Why some people become mentally ill and not others, and why some people become mentally ill at some periods in their lives, but at other times seem to take major stresses in their stride, is even less understood than the causes of physical illnesses. Although some researchers and clinicians still take the view that mental disorders are either entirely caused by biological factors (physical diseases of the brain), or entirely caused by purely psychological factors, the consensus of professional thinking tends towards assuming that some combination of these factors is responsible.

> *Theories about causes … and proposals for treatment can be grouped under one of the following perspectives: biological, psychoanalytic, behavioural and cognitive. The vulnerability–stress model emphasises the interaction between a predisposition (biological and/or psychological) that makes a person vulnerable for developing a disorder and stressful environmental conditions that the individual encounters.*
>
> Atkinson *et al.* 1996, p. 515

Some illnesses, particularly of a schizophrenic type, can have a very slow, insidious onset, seemingly unrelated to any obvious crisis. Schizophrenia is typically an illness of late adolescence, a time when the individual personality is seeking to progressively assert greater independence and autonomy. This, for some people, might be experienced as a prolonged period of both interpersonal and intrapersonal maturational stress.

This is the context in which the following stories are set. Each person featured, while suffering from a form of mental illness, is subject to the infinitely variable range of stresses and stressors mentioned above. The stories do not, and could not, cover the whole spectrum of mental illness. They illustrate how the skills, techniques and ideas discussed in the previous chapters could be used in a limited range of situations.

5.2 PREAMBLE, PROFILE, PATHWAY, PROGNOSIS

The following stories set a range of mental illnesses and disorders into hospital, day hospital and social settings so that the difficulties are rightly seen as they impact on other people, not just on the patient/client and the nurse. You will also see how the person's environment influences the way they manage (or don't manage) their illness. From this you will see that to nurse any person fully, holistically and effectively it is essential to try to take into account:

- *Their significant others.* Parents, siblings, relatives, friends, neighbours may all have an impact or influence, historically, immediately, or in the future. Significant others who are dead may also need to be taken into consideration. For example you will find the people you meet may not necessarily have positive relationships with their parents, their children, or their siblings. They may have feelings of antipathy or ambivalence towards dead relations. You will notice that some people you meet who have the role of 'patient' seem to be socially isolated or alone.

Discussion point

What could be some of the reasons for this?

Be careful not to assume that the quality of the relationships between family members is some kind of replica of your own. You may even at some point, when talking with relatives, ponder why it is that they seem to be needier than your patient/client.

Discussion point

How is it that the person in your care has taken on or been given the role of the 'patient' while other members of the family survive outside the mental health services?

A genogram can be very helpful to you when you are trying to make sense of all this (see section 3.9).

- *Their environment.* This includes their housing circumstances, the area where they live, the cultures that exist in that area. For example, does the patient live in a white middle-class area where the neighbours are prosperous, or do they live in a inner-city or suburban deprived area where many of their neighbours are unable to find work?

Discussion point

Taking into account your subjective anecdotal experience, which of the above two categories do most of your patients and clients fall into ... or do they fall into some other category? Why is it sometimes possible to categorise patients into groups? What does this achieve?

- *Other aspects.* The person's aspirations, fears, wishes, spiritual position or secular beliefs (they may be lost in respect of this). For example, some patients and clients do not seem to have any religious belief. On the other hand a small number have an almost overwhelming religious belief. You will find that sometimes any sense of ambition, drive or feeling for a positive future is missing. Clients may have a disproportionate fear of something that is a threat to us all but their fear is many times magnified. Any new media-reported epidemic, for instance, such as the SARS episode in the early 2000s or HIV/AIDS in the 1980s is often focused on by people who are prone to psychosis (delusions of reference; Bloye and Davies 1999).

Discussion point

Why are strongly held religious views often a focus of intense distress or grandiose delusions in some mentally ill people?

Preamble

Before each story the background of the illness will be briefly explored as it is generally understood. For greater depth, go to any of the many basic mental health texts listed in the reference section.

Profile

The person will be sketched out in terms of their general characteristics and background. This will model how you might present a new patient or client to the care team, so that your colleagues can quickly construct a mental picture of the new person.

The reasons you may be expected to do this are several:

- *You are the client's named (associate) nurse.* Therefore you are the person who is going to be the first point of contact for many enquiries about that patient/client. In this sense you become an 'expert' and advocate in terms of your level of knowledge about the situation of this patient. If you feel that you are not, then try to identify the factors that are stopping you from being an expert and try to address them.
- *You are the person who carried out the client's initial assessment.* You will have seen the person at the point of, or very near to, their admission. It is likely that their presentation will change as time goes on but nevertheless the information given by the person at admission is essential to start to formulate an initial care plan.
- *You are the person to whom that client seems to relate best.* There is sometimes no easy explanation as to why this happens. It might be to do with your age, your gender, the way you look, the way you are.

A patient/client profile should be presented in a structured, easy-to-follow, methodical way that is logical and that makes sense to you. For example:

- Name
- Age
- Reason for referral or admission
- Background (e.g. locality, occupation, family) – if there isn't a set format given to you by your team, you will gradually develop a systematic way of doing this)
- Results of your assessment, preferably using appropriate evidence-based systems wherever possible.

Pathway or route

This means the pathway or route from the onset of the difficulties through to the point of discharge/referral. Assessment, planning and implementing of care, and evaluating the effectiveness of the care will be tracked. The different carers (formal and informal) and range of professionals who may be involved will be described. An attempt has been made with all of these processes to capture the sometimes extremely difficult nature of mental health nursing, in which patience and consistency are invaluable personal attributes.

Prognosis

The likely range of possible resolutions from the ending of the pathway/route explored. In mental illness there often isn't a happy ending.

5.3 ACUTE DEPRESSION WITH ANXIETY – JOANNE

Preamble

Depression is probably the most common mental illness. Most people have some idea of what it is to be low in mood or spirit. Not as many people know what it is like to feel so hopeless that they would like to stop living. Many people who experience moods that are this severe feel a kind of ambivalence towards their own life (Cardell and Horton-Deutsch 1994, Thompson 1999). You may hear them say things like 'I wish I could go to sleep and not wake up' or ' If there was a pill I could take to just end my life, I'd take it'. Others say that the only reason that they don't kill themselves is because of the pain that it would cause to others, especially their children. Of course, some people go even beyond this reasoning and attempt to end their lives regardless of the survivors. Traditionally, males seem to choose more violent and irreversible methods, while females tend to choose ways that are more passive and in some ways less absolute (Bergman 1991, Clark 1992, Stuart and Laraia 2001).

The treatments have not changed radically for many years. A relatively recent change in treatment style is the uptake of cognitive and cognitive behavioural (CBT) approaches by many practitioners (not only for depressive illnesses – see Chapter 1).

Antidepressants have some history of success but don't work for everyone (Fredman *et al.* 2000, Parker and Roy 2001). The latest generation of anti-depressants is called selective serotonin re-uptake inhibitors (SSRIs). At the time of writing there are doubts being expressed about the effectiveness of this group of drugs (Prabhakaran 2002, Opbrock 2002). Historically, doubts have been expressed about many groups of drugs and will continue to be so (Stuart and Laraia 2001.

Electroconvulsive therapy (ECT) is also used on a widespread basis despite some people's feeling that it is an unethical form of treatment (Stuart and Laraia 2001). It does seem to lift the depressed mood of some people – but again, not all of them. This highlights a characteristic of depression – that no one treatment is effective for all sufferers.

Over time the treatment that seems to work for many people is a combination of a 'talking therapy' (cognitive therapy, counselling, psychotherapy and so on) and an appropriate dose of one of the antidepressants. There are some indications that depression will occasionally resolve of its own accord anyway (Nierenberg 2001).

The impact of depression on the new generation of mental health carers is not to be underestimated. The World Health Organization suggests that the epidemic of this millennium will be depression and melancholia (Barker 1999).

A proportion of depression sufferers also have problems with periods of anxiety. Anxiety is an emotion that is associated with the perception of possible or actual threat. It may not always be an entirely negative emotion, since some of the physical symptoms (see below) are also characteristic of excitement or pleasurable anticipation. It is a normal emotion, without which we would lack motivation to avoid danger or to make particular effort to perform on special occasions. But anxiety can also become abnormal or disproportionate in intensity, sometimes persistently so. It is then that it may be described as a clinical anxiety state, which may respond positively to professional help.

Over the years, psychiatrists and psychologists have divided abnormal anxiety into a number of specific subcategories, which may occur as distinct syndromes but frequently overlap and merge with each other. Current classifications recognise 'general anxiety', 'phobic anxiety' and 'panic attacks', but other syndromes such as obsessive–compulsive disorder and obsessional slowness are also regarded as being forms of anxiety state, or rather, extreme defence mechanisms against it.

As patients and clients rarely fall into neatly defined textbook categories, this first story will consider an ambiguous hypothetical 'case-study', representing a mix of symptoms and problems. It should be emphasised that, as well as being recognised as a cluster of conditions in its own right, marked anxiety can frequently be a component of almost any other form of mental health diagnosis or psychological distress. Depression and anxiety are often inextricably linked and mutually reinforcing. Therefore, the examples, strategies and skills described in this chapter serve to illustrate some of the ways in which people like Joanne can be helped by mental health carers.

Profile

Joanne's referral letter from the GP to the Community Mental Health Trust stated that she was a 31-year-old woman, married with two young children. She had been experiencing panic attacks since a few weeks after the birth of her second child, just over a year ago. Over the last two or three months the attacks had been getting more frequent and she was becoming increasingly reluctant to leave the house.

Discussion point

How would you present this profile in a team meeting? What other things are the team likely to want to know about Joanne?

Pathway through the disorder

Two weeks after receiving the referral, Community Psychiatric Nurse Ruth Simpson was making her first visit to see Joanne at her home for an initial assessment. Ruth had initially written to Joanne to inform her of her wish to visit, and the date and time had been negotiated by phone. Ruth was accompanied by student nurse Sharon Green.

This was Sharon's second week of community nursing experience. Now in her second year of training, she had already completed two 'inpatient' placements and one in a day hospital. She had accompanied Ruth on a few visits already, to see established clients on her case-load, but this was her first chance to participate in an initial assessment.

En route to the appointment Sharon enquired about Ruth's expectations of her as an inexperienced student in this situation. It was agreed that Sharon was there primarily as an observer but that it might create a rather difficult atmosphere if Sharon did not feel able to contribute verbally to the interaction beyond the first introductions. Ruth suggested that Sharon should have some confidence in her own judgement about what she should say and when, but to keep her responses briefly empathic or politely neutral. Respectfully attentive non-verbal behaviour would probably be the client's primary need from Sharon on this occasion. When Sharon asked Ruth what she meant by this, Ruth explained: 'Try to show that you're interested. Ask a few questions if you like, but think what you're doing. If in doubt, shut up. Give Mrs Fraser some non-verbal encouragement. Little nods to affirm what she says are useful. Don't stare at her. Keep breaking off your eye contact. Be friendly. Smile a bit. That'll do to start with.'

The house was semi-detached with a small front garden, situated in a quiet suburban street. They were only kept waiting a few seconds on the doorstep. As the door opened Sharon observed a fair haired young woman of slim build and tidy appearance, who smiled at them in greeting. Ruth is the first to speak:

Ruth. Hello. Mrs Joanne Fraser? (*It is important, for confidentiality reasons, for Ruth to check that she is speaking to the client before explaining exactly who she is.*) Hi – I'm Ruth Simpson, the community nurse (*she deliberately doesn't say 'psychiatric nurse'. She is aware of the stigma associated with this term*). We spoke on the phone the other day. This is Sharon, the student I told you about.

Sharon smiles and says 'Hello'. She notices that Joanne acknowledges her greeting with brief eye contact and a rather more hesitant smile. She shows them into a through lounge. An older woman is in the process of securing a young child into a push-chair.

Linda. Hello, I'm Linda, Joanne's mum.

She explains that she is just about to take the baby out for a walk, so that they can talk to Joanne without interruption.

Linda. I'm so glad you're here. We've been waiting so long for some help for Joanne.

Joanne herself is starting to look more hesitant and uncomfortable in manner.

Joanne. Won't you sit down? Just let me tidy these toys up. Would you like a cup of tea or coffee?

Both nurses accept the offer. Ruth has explained to Sharon earlier that she usually prefers not to accept a drink at the first visit, as the delay of making it can sometimes prolong the awkwardness at the start of the first meeting, although she acknowledges that it can also help to 'normalise' the situation and decrease the formality. Ruth smiles broadly at the child in the push-chair:

Ruth. What a beautiful little girl. Are you going to take Grandma for a nice walk? (*The use of gentle, appropriate humour can be useful, even in very tense situations. The intention is always to help the client.*)

Joanne looks at Ruth:

Joanne. You didn't say how long you wanted to talk to me. Oh, I feel so foolish.

She gives a half sob, and her breathing is becoming noticeably shallower and more rapid. She puts her hand to her forehead and partially covers her face. Her other hand clenches at her side.

Ruth. I usually expect to take just over an hour for a first meeting.

Ruth starts to explain in a deliberately calm tone of voice but it is obvious that Joanne is no longer really paying attention. Her breathing is faster than ever, one hand is clutched to her chest and with the other she is tightly gripping the back of a chair. Her face looks anguished and her voice rises:

Joanne. Oh, I can't stand these feelings all the time, I can't stand them! Why won't they stop? What can I do?'

Joanne is hyperventilating and sobbing at the same time. She says her heart is beating so much it feels like it's going to burst out of her chest and she can't stand the sound of the baby crying.

Ruth has moved slightly closer to Joanne now and is facing her, seeking eye contact. She looks concerned but is composed in manner. Speaking very clearly, so as to be heard above the sound of the baby crying, she talks directly to Joanne, in an even, sympathetic, but also a quite 'matter of fact' tone of voice:

> **Ruth.** Joanne, what you're feeling now is horrible and maybe quite scary. I suspect it's been happening to you a lot just lately. What do you want your Mum to do? Do you want her to still take the baby out as planned? (*This is an early attempt to show empathy with the client and some evidence that the nurse has some inkling of what the person is going through.*)
> **Joanne.** I don't know. I don't know what to do – I never know what to do. I feel so frightened all the time. I can't cope.

Still in the same even, clear tone, Ruth asks her if she wants to pick the baby up to comfort her:

> **Joanne.** No, no, I can't, I'm no good to her like this, I'll make her worse. If I faint I might drop her!
> **Ruth.** Well then, can I suggest that your Mum takes the baby out for half an hour at least, and see if that settles her down, while you and I have a chat?
> **Joanne.** I can't talk like this, I can't. Oh, you can see I'm in no state to talk, this is all a mistake, you won't be able to help me, the doctors won't help me, they don't understand, they just keep saying there's nothing physically wrong with me, but it's not normal to be like this, I just want it to stop.
> **Ruth.** I think I can help you Joanne, if you'll give me a chance to try. (*She puts her hand on Joanne's arm at this point and continues to speak firmly, but kindly, with just a trace of humour in her voice.*) I don't want to give up before I've even started.

Sharon notices that Joanne's mother is looking at Ruth now as though she has a bit of confidence in her. She opens the door to the hallway and announces that she will take the baby for a walk to calm her down, and give them all some time to talk. 'I'll come back in about an hour, if that's OK.'

> **Ruth.** Thanks, that will be just fine, I think.
> **Joanne.** You must think I'm a useless mother – she only got so upset because of me, I just upset everyone, I'm going mad, I know I am, I'll never be normal!'
> **Ruth.** Joanne, would you like Sharon to get you a glass of water?
> **Joanne** nods in reply.

Sharon returns a minute later with the glass of water, to find Ruth still standing patiently beside Joanne, calmly accepting. Ruth takes the glass of water from Sharon, and offers it to Joanne.

> **Ruth.** Try and have a sip. Do you think you could sit down?

Joanne nods as she takes the water from her and moves to sit tensely on the edge of one of the armchairs, her eyes focused on the floor. She glances towards Ruth's face, after taking another sip of water:

Joanne. I can still feel it here.

She touches her chest with her other hand. Her breathing is still rapid and shallow but perhaps not quite as much so as a couple of minutes ago.

Ruth. Is there anything you've tried that makes it a bit easier to tolerate?

Joanne shakes her head dismissively. Her hyperventilating seems to be happening again. Sharon tries to count Joanne's respirations, which she estimates at about 120 a minute.

Joanne. No – the practice nurse at the doctor's gave me a . . . 'relaxation tape' she called it. It didn't help. I listened to it a few times and tried to follow the instructions. I couldn't stand the condescending tone of the woman's voice. I tried it again the other day, but it's still no good. You can see the state I'm in. I bet you think I'm really silly don't you?

Ruth. No, I think you are unwell, you are obviously having a real struggle coping with it, and there's nothing silly about that. Can I suggest something? Your breathing is very rapid and shallow at the moment, because of your anxiety, but it's also maintaining all the other feelings like your heart thumping. Some people find it helps to breathe in and out of their cupped hands, or a paper bag. Have you ever tried that? It will help a little.

This is expert advice that may help to decrease the distressing physical symptoms a little more quickly. Although she looks unconvinced by the advice, Joanne does as she is asked, sitting with her elbows on her knees, and her hands cupped round her mouth. Ruth explains that hyperventilation (over-breathing) causes a 'vicious circle' of worsening symptoms due to the loss of too much carbon dioxide. She also points out to Joanne that her body looks very tense. She tells her that the feelings she is having may subside faster if she can relax some of her muscles. She briefly gives her some simple instructions to try and follow.

Joanne is exhibiting many of the signs of a typical 'panic attack', described in the DSM-IV manual as a 'discrete period of intense discomfort' in which several physical and psychological symptoms of extreme anxiety develop abruptly and reach a peak within a few minutes. It is often a sudden wave of overwhelming fear and terror, accompanied by physical sensations of rapid, bounding heartbeat and a feeling of impending collapse, or choking and suffocation. These attacks can occur without any obvious precipitating event or in response to a general fear of not being able to cope with a particular situation. Such episodes usually subside in intensity within minutes rather than hours, although many sufferers continue to experience varying degrees of anxiety between attacks. Occasional episodes of extreme anxiety or panic are said to be common in the general population.

Newell and Gournay (2000) observe that most nurses will encounter a patient/ client with a panic attack early in their career and offer some simple rules for how they might be managed. They state that panic attacks do not lead to death or heart attacks. However, it is essential to know that patients have been screened thoroughly by a doctor to eliminate the possibility of heart disease or endocrine disorders. Many patients find it difficult to accept even repeated medical reassurances that there is nothing physically wrong with them, like

Joanne, but even if they do, such knowledge is not usually sufficient to prevent repeated attacks.

It is generally agreed that the nurse should appear calm and unflustered herself. Patients and bystanders are best reassured by the nurse maintaining an appearance of confident self-control while giving simple instructions in a low, relaxed voice (Gournay 2003). Patients should be encouraged to sit or lie down and stay as still as possible. They should also be asked to try and slow their breathing by breathing from the diaphragm. It is often most effective if the nurse demonstrates this by placing a hand on his/her own abdomen and showing the breathing in a slightly over-exaggerated way, to make clear what is happening.

Ruth does not offer Joanne any reassurance that she is not going to have a heart attack. This is a very common preoccupation of panic attack sufferers and many textbooks emphasise the need for such reassurance. However, Joanne has not actually expressed the fear on this occasion and Ruth makes the judgement that it might be patronising to give such assurances. Joanne has been experiencing such feelings for at least some months and has discussed them with her doctor on more than one occasion. Ruth's primary aim is to caringly communicate an expectation that the feelings will subside more quickly if they are not over-reacted to, and at the same time to prompt Joanne to do some practical things that will help her exercise some control.

After a while, Joanne is starting to appear a little more composed. Ruth asks her if she would like a little fresh air, and suggests going into the garden for a few minutes. Joanne seems to welcome this suggestion. She stands at the kitchen door but says she doesn't want to go out in the garden, as she doesn't know how she will introduce Ruth and Sharon to the neighbours if they are outside as well.

Joanne. Do you think I should take a tablet?

She explains that her doctor prescribed her some Valium. She knows about the risks of dependency but says that she cannot manage without it, especially first thing in the morning when she has to get Michael ready for school. Then she corrects herself, saying:

It's Simon who gets him ready, really, while I look after Lucy until my mother gets here. If I didn't have a tablet in the morning I'd get all panicky when it's time for him to leave the house and go to school. It's hard enough anyway.

She goes silent and just seems content to stand for a while looking down the garden. She seems to have forgotten about taking a tablet.

Now that Joanne seems to have composed herself a little more, Ruth asks if they can go back in and talk about what's been happening. Joanne offers them a cup of coffee again (could caffeine have anything to do with her anxiety? See Jacobson and Jacobson 1996) but Ruth declines, saying she would rather Joanne used the time before her mum returns with Lucy to talk in as much detail as she feels able to.

Joanne. Yes, all right.

She tries to take a deep breath but she is still obviously very tense, and Sharon notices she is trembling slightly.

They return to the lounge and sit down. Ruth sits a little further away from her now, because the proxemics are critical here. Joanne mustn't feel crowded or pushed. Ruth's attention to this helps Joanne's feelings of being in control of her situation as much as possible.

Although when people are in a state of extreme distress, such as a panic attack, the close physical presence of an empathic nurse may be reassuring, the nurse also needs to respect the client's need for personal space. Stuart and Laraia (2001, p. 25) quote research by Brown and Yantis (1996), which suggests that 'a 6 foot distance in a small room may create the optimum condition for openness and discussion of fears. The more this distance is increased or decreased, the more anxious a patient may become.' It will not always be practical to observe these limits precisely, and they will vary in significance from one individual to another. However, the research is cited as a reminder of the importance of not taking trust for granted. It has to be earned. Establishing a therapeutic relationship takes time and commitment. Sensitivity to spatial proximity is just one of many factors that contributes to creating a feeling of psychological security.

Ruth summarises the information contained in the GP's referral letter, but says she would like to hear Joanne's account in her own words.

> **Ruth.** When do you think things started to go wrong?
> **Joanne.** Oh, it all seems to have been going on so long. I don't really know what caused it. I've always been rather a nervous person, but I started to feel worse after Lucy was born.
> I was so looking forward to having this second baby. Michael is our eldest; he's just started school a few weeks ago. He'll be coming home for lunch in just over an hour. I miss him when he's not here.
> It wasn't an easy time around the period he was born. My father was diagnosed with cancer just after I found out I was pregnant, and he died before Michael was 2 months old. He would have made a lovely grandad. At least he saw him.

Joanne's eyes are filling with tears as she speaks (a catharsis is happening – Ruth has to decide whether to encourage it or dampen it). Ruth, who is sitting slightly diagonally to Joanne, says nothing, but her body is turned towards her, leaning slightly forward, and she is clearly giving Joanne her full attention.

Joanne is silently weeping now. Without changing her posture, in a soft but clear voice, Ruth simply acknowledges what Joanne is feeling:

> **Ruth.** That's very sad.

By encouraging the expression of strong emotion, avoiding comforting or diverting attention from the feeling, and by initially remaining silent when Joanne was starting to feel upset, Ruth may have helped the feeling to fully surface.

Joanne dabs her eyes with the back of her hand. Her nose is running slightly and she sniffs to try and control it. Sharon remembers noticing there were some tissues on a shelf in the corner and asks 'Can we use these?' (Again demonstrating respect for Joanne's property and territory).

> Joanne. I still can't talk about Dad's death in front of Mum. He was only 58 when he died. She still gets upset at the mention of his name. We called Michael after him.

Joanne goes on to explain the events of their lives since that time. She talks freely now, with little need for any prompting or responses from Ruth.

However, after about 20 minutes, Ruth – who has not been taking notes – takes advantage of a natural pause in Joanne's narrative to summarise (see also section 2.20) what she has heard and attempt to empathise with Joanne:

> Ruth. So, what should have been a time of happiness and joy at the birth of your son was mixed with grief for your father?
>
> Joanne. Yes, we were happy about Michael – he was a lovely baby, he's a lovely little boy, but I did feel guilty about being so thrilled about him when I should have been feeling sad about my Dad. I mean I *was* sad about Dad, of course I was, but it was so difficult having both sets of feelings at once. Dad didn't want us to be sad, he tried so hard to make things easier for us.
>
> Ruth. But it's been hard for your mum as well. You've been worried about her as well, and perhaps you were not always able to share your joy in the birth of your son as much as you needed to?'
>
> Joanne. I don't know. Mum was as proud of him as I was. I don't think that was the problem. It was not being able to talk about Dad, and how much Michael would miss out by not knowing his grandad. I couldn't talk about that. I couldn't even talk about how much I missed him.

Joanne is starting to look tearful again, but does not break down.

> Ruth. You said you had a friend who suffered from anxiety and depression and you recognised you had some of the same symptoms as her. But you didn't feel depressed, you said. Worried about your mum and still sad about your dad, but not depressed. You extended your maternity leave but when you did go back to work the panic attacks became really severe and you had to get someone to take you home. You were off sick for nearly two months, then things seemed a bit better and you were able to return to work, but then they started again about two months ago and now you've been off sick again for nearly a month. You've had a tough time, haven't you?
>
> Joanne. But you must see people with far worse problems. I worry that people will think I'm just being a fraud, and yet I can't help it. I feel so out of control.
>
> Ruth. That doesn't sound like someone who's being a fraud. Do you ever feel that you can't go on? That it's too much to bear?
>
> Joanne. Sometimes.
>
> Ruth. What do you think of doing at those times? (*Ruth is now probing for possible suicidal intent.*)
>
> Joanne. I just wish I could go to sleep and not wake up. But then other times I think I should feel grateful for two lovely children. I can't bear the thought that I wouldn't see them again.
>
> Ruth. I'm not sure I 'm understanding you. Why wouldn't you see them again?'
>
> Joanne. If I went to sleep and didn't wake up again I mean.
>
> Ruth. Do you ever feel you could do anything to make that happen?
>
> Joanne. Take an overdose, you mean? Dr Jones asked me that. I couldn't do it.

It wouldn't be fair on Simon or the children or anyone. No I've never felt that bad, I don't think. Did you think I had?

Ruth. We have to ask about these things. Some people do feel very desperate sometimes. If we don't ask we don't always find out how they are. It's better to be able to talk about such feelings and thoughts. Joanne, I noticed that you've not talked much about Simon. What's been his reaction?'

Ruth is now wanting to make some appraisal of the strength of the marital relationship and whether Joanne sees her husband as supportive or otherwise.

It should be noted that her questions are timed and phrased in response to cues from Joanne herself. Joanne had just introduced her husband into the conversation. A little earlier when Ruth had asked about whether Joanne ever felt that she couldn't carry on any longer, this was prompted by Joanne's statement that she 'felt so out of control'.

The timing of these more closed questions demonstrates the principle of immediacy (Stuart and Laraia 2001), as well as client-centredness (Rogers 1951). Ruth knows the important assessment criteria she has to seek information about, but she does not want her need for information to inhibit spontaneous self-disclosure from Joanne by asking too many closed questions in a pre-set order. Because of her experience, Ruth is working systematically through a list of criteria, but Joanne is unaware of this. To her it seems like a conversation.

Joanne. Oh, he's been very tolerant. Too tolerant sometimes. I know it gets him down. I feel guilty about that as well

Ruth. Is there any particular time when things seem worse than usual?

Joanne. In the mornings when Simon leaves for work and Michael goes to school. Sometimes Simon takes him and drops him off, sometimes Mum comes round and takes him. When I see them leave I start to imagine all sorts of horrible things happening to them. Sometimes I know it's stupid, but I can't stop the thoughts. Some of the things are horrible.

Ruth. Your mum will be home soon, with Lucy. You might not feel able to talk so freely then. We've got a few minutes in which I 'd like to clarify a few more points and make some suggestions.

I'd like to see you again if you think it will do any good. How about coming to our base to see how it is talking with us in a different environment? We could use a room at your GP's?

Joanne. What if I can't get there, though? I've not been out of the house on my own for weeks.

Ruth. Which day would be convenient for you?

Ruth delays responding to Joanne's question. She has recognised that Joanne is displaying what behaviourists term simultaneous 'approach–avoidance' feelings (Stuart and Laraia 2001). She has expressed a wish to talk to Ruth again in a more private setting where she will not be distracted by her baby or possibly inhibited by her mum's presence. But she has apparently established a pattern of rarely or never leaving the house to go anywhere on her own. Ruth is hoping that, if she doesn't give her any immediate avoidance option, her motivation to attend the meeting at the GP's clinic will be strengthened. This could be regarded as a small, calculated, therapeutic risk.

> Ruth. One of us will be there waiting. Is it all right if Sharon joins us again?
> Joanne. Oh yes, I don't mind. Of course she can. It helps a little somehow, being with both of you. Thank you. I'm starting to feel calmer now

Joanne might also be starting to feel calmer because she knows the meeting is coming to an end and it is nearly time for the two nurses to leave.

> Ruth. Is there anything you would like to ask us before we leave?
> Joanne. Do you think I'll ever be any better?
> Ruth. I hope so. I think talking about that might be a good place for us to start on Thursday.

Summary of communication skills used

- Consistent
- Reassuring
- Honest
- Empathic
- Open questions
- Directive when appropriate
- Clear, regarding intentions
- Tentative
- Approachable
- Working towards therapeutic relationship
- Empowering
- Good listener
- Intuitive
- Aware of boundaries and finishing
- Using touch if appropriate
- Using humour when appropriate.

Summary of approaches that make up the strategy

Ruth's strategy is first to try to create a trusting rapport. Once this is begun she can begin to effectively assess. Her initial intentions are to inform, support and assess. They will be closely followed by the need to obtain information and encourage expression of feelings. She will be aware that the relationship is time-limited, and she makes this clear to her client. She works collaboratively with other members of her care team. She tries to involve her client in any plan of care. She notes the relationships that are important to her client and takes these into account when assessing and implementing treatment.

Prognosis

A future goal would be for Ruth to speak at greater length with Joanne's mother, Linda, and also with her husband, Simon – with, of course, Joanne's permission.

The original referral from the GP indicated a case of an apparently socially isolated young woman who had developed an anxiety state, with episodes of panic and an increasing tendency to agoraphobia, with perhaps a tendency to slip towards depression.

The vast majority of nursing textbooks published in the last 10 years would have advocated a behaviour-oriented strategy of anxiety management, including patient education about the effects of anxiety creating a 'vicious circle' of escalating symptoms unless the cycle is broken. This would be combined with practical instruction on breathing exercises, relaxation therapy (deep muscle relaxation), possibly graduated exposure to avoided situations (ideally under the supervision of a specialist behaviour therapist), probably coupled with cognitive interventions to challenge a tendency to 'catastrophise' (Gelder *et al* 1999) any perception of potential risk (see also CBT approach).

All of the above may be helpful to Joanne but the presenting picture suggests more complex needs and risks. This may not be the last time that Joanne seeks professional mental health support. The ways that Ruth has shown her to manage her problems need reinforcing and encouragement from a supportive and approachable carer, otherwise there is a danger that all the good work will erode. Coming from the psychologically defeated position of Joanne it is not unusual for sufferers to become despondent and once again experience a spiralling down of mood.

The likelihood is that Joanne will recover, as long as the support she gets from professional carers and her family is consistent. She may feel fragile for some time but there is no evidence that she is doomed to relapse.

5.4 LONGER-TERM DEPRESSION – JON

Preamble

The DSM-IV differentiates between Major Depressive Disorders (American Psychiatric Association 1994, p. 339) and Dysthymia (p. 345) by comparing 'severity, chronicity, and persistence' (p. 343). When assessing people who may be suffering from low mood, it is prudent to make sure that they are experiencing an established cluster of symptoms before rushing into an assumption that the person before you is depressed. They may be going through a 'bad patch' or they may be suffering a drop in mood that will pass.

It is important to see if there is any such history of patterns, as some people seem to suffer from this as part of the pathology of their personality. It doesn't necessarily indicate that they are mentally ill. They may be the victims of what used to be commonly known as 'melancholia' (Jacobson and Jacobson 1996).

When assessing, it may be helpful to look out for significant dates, such as the anniversaries of losses that are important to the person. Be careful about making assumptions here. What you might think should be an important loss may not be, and *vice versa*. A person may feel that the death of Elvis, or their cat, is more important to them than the death of their parent. On the other hand, some people can seem to manage multiple losses that would seem very significant, and still get through without becoming overwhelmed by a clinical depression.

Varcarolis (2000, p. 163) lists some useful sample questions such as: 'When you get sad or down how long does it last? …What do you see for yourself in the future?' Also, she notes that more objective tests such as the Beck Depression Inventory can be used to assess. Perhaps it does not matter too much which model or theories form the basis of your own key beliefs about the causes of depression. You may believe that it is anger turned inwards (Thomas *et al.* 1998,

p. 355), the result of negative cognitions (p. 356) or learned behaviours (p. 357). Whatever your belief(s) the assessment approach you use can still be based on the rudiments in this book.

Profile

Jon is a 43-year-old man who has been married to Jenny for 15 years. They have two sons, Daniel who is 12 and Chris who is 7. They all live in a four-bedroom detached house on the outskirts of a large Midlands city. Jon works as a design engineer in an independent engineering company. He has done this for the past 12 years. Jenny is a supply teacher.

Discussion point

The style of presentation of information in the above section would provide a useful template for any briefing that you do either to a single colleague or within a group meeting such as a care review or a shift handover. Laying out the objective data about a person helps others 'set the scene' in their heads. It doesn't matter if you think everyone in the room is familiar with all this information, there may be someone who isn't, or there may be someone who has missed part of it. Occasionally you will find that a brief recap also helps reveal aspects of the person's situation that perhaps weren't at first apparent.

Daniel is doing well at school. His teachers describe him as an exemplary pupil. Chris is more boisterous and his teacher describes him as 'a handful sometimes'. Jon's mother has recently been taken into a care home after a stroke. She seems to not recognise any of the family when they visit her. Jenny's parents both died when she was young.

Recently, she notices, Jon has been working very late on 'projects'. She notices also that he doesn't seem to be bothered about the way he looks any more. Previously he was 'almost obsessive' (she says) about his appearance. They seem to be having rows that are much more 'bitter' and longer-lasting than previously. They have always argued but somehow, to Jenny, this feels different.

One morning after a particularly bad row she says, partially in temper: 'Why don't you go to the doctor? You're bloody depressed.' She is surprised to hear herself saying this. Jon looks shaken.

Discussion point

There is a range of losses for both Jon and Jenny and their children. What are they? Is there any significance in the ages of the family members, the occupations that Jon and Jenny have, the length of their relationship, the place they live, their choice of house? What is the significance of Jon's projects? What might Jenny mean when she uses language like 'almost obsessive ... depressed ... bitter'? How has the nature of their arguments altered? What may have caused Jon to lose interest in his appearance?

Pathway through depression

Jon visits his GP's surgery.

Dr Stevens. How can I help?
Jon. My wife thinks I'm depressed
Dr Stevens. Why do you think she says that?
Jon. I don't know. We've argued a lot lately. I've a lot on my mind.

They talk for about 10 minutes. Jon gives the impression that he doesn't really understand what is happening to him. He's just doing this 'to keep his wife quiet'. Certainly, Dr Stevens picks up a few things about Jon that might indicate a mild depression or dysthymia. He seems to have difficulty getting to sleep, regardless of how tired he is. At around 5 o'clock every morning, without fail, he wakes up. He then can't get to sleep again until just before the alarm goes off at 7.30. He doesn't feel hungry and usually makes himself a sandwich when he gets in from work. By this time Jenny is helping the boys get ready for bed. Their sex life is non-existent. Jon never feels like it and Jenny is always fast asleep anyway.

Objectively Dr Stevens thinks that Jon is showing a small cluster of symptoms that seem to indicate a dysthymic episode. The length of time that Jon seems to have been suffering lends weight to this hypothesis. Subjectively Dr Stevens feels that something else is not quite right. It's something to do with the way Jon refers to his wife. He thinks that maybe, if antidepressants don't seem to have any impact, he'll consider the practice counsellor or the community mental health team.

Dr Stevens decides to prescribe a course of antidepressants as a first attempt to help Jon:

Dr Stevens. If you start to feel worse, come back and see me. Whatever happens, come back and see me in two weeks. Give them a chance, though, they may take two or three weeks before you start to feel any better.

Seven weeks later, after a couple of monitoring visits, Jon returns to the surgery:

Jon. Those tablets you gave me aren't doing anything. I feel worse. I keep thinking that I can't go to work anymore. We're having terrible rows. I don't know what to do. I feel worse than I have ever felt in my entire life – worn out, beaten – lost, really.

Discussion point

If Jon used these words in conversation with you, how might you respond? Look at the use of his language. What does he actually mean by the use of this imagery in his language?

Dr Stevens decides to refer him to the local community mental health team. Two weeks later, after phoning to make an appointment, the community psychiatric nurse allocated to assess him arrives at Jon's home.

Nicola. Hi, I'm Nicola, the Community Nurse. We spoke on the phone a couple of days ago?

Nicola starts an assessment, which will last about an hour. Her plan is to then present her findings to her colleagues at a weekly multi-disciplinary meeting to decide:

- Has Jon a treatable mental illness?
- Is he suitable for treatment by the team?
- Who will help him
- When/how will they do it?

> Nicola. The letter that Dr Stevens sent the team mentioned that you were struggling with sleep as well as some other issues. Could you talk me through what's happening at the moment?

Notice the tentative style used by Nicola, even when first meeting Jon at the doorstep. She avoids using the terms 'psychiatric' or 'mental health' when she introduces herself. She is acutely aware that at this stage she needs to reduce, or keep at a minimum any resistance (Stuart and Laraia 2001) in her 'client'. She is surprised to see Jenny, Jon's wife, at the meeting. She wasn't expecting this (Jenny has taken the day off work to be present when Nicola calls to see Jon). Therefore, her approach is that of giving minimal information away in front of Jenny. It is not clear yet how much Jenny knows and, again, Nicola does not want to endanger the relationship she has already started with Jon (she did this from the point of the original phone call, to confirm their meeting) by appearing to encroach on his privacy.

Hence, Nicola refers to the GP's letter in as little detail as possible and uses Jon's lack of sleep as a starter topic, as it is a relatively safe area to discuss in front of Jenny, given that she is not sure yet how welcoming Jon will be towards her.

> Jon. Yeah, it's no better … although I'm off work now, so it doesn't matter so much.
> Jenny. Are you going to tell Nicola about throwing the tablets away? That really helped, didn't it?

Already, with just one careful question, Nicola becomes quickly aware of several vital pieces of information:

- Jon's sleep remains apparently troubled
- He is now unable or unwilling to go to work
- He was not compliant in taking the prescribed medication
- His wife is aggressive towards him at the moment.

You will see that this is some of the data from one thoughtfully phrased question. It is now up to Nicola to quickly decide which of these pieces of information she wishes to pursue. Her decision will be influenced by a combination of wanting to develop perhaps the most powerfully influential of these choices.

Discussion point

Which one would you choose in this situation? What could be the significance of the other choices?

Whatever she decides, it is very likely that she will return to each topic in the future (see also section 2.13). That could be in the next few minutes, before the end of this assessment meeting or in future meetings. She decides at this moment to pursue the angle of Jon's non-compliance regarding his prescribed medication.

Nicola. Jon, what was behind your decision to stop taking the medication that your GP suggested?

Jon. Nothing was happening. I took them every day for about four weeks. I read the leaflet in the packet on side effects . . . it's horrifying. A friend at work said that his father had them and they made him worse. I put them down the toilet.

Jenny. Good one. Could you sort him out? He's driving me crackers always slouched around at home. Even the boys are getting fed up with him. Why don't you get your act together and go back to work?

Nicola avoids becoming entangled in the apparent conflict between Jon and Jenny. She suggests that Jon completes a couple of questionnaires so that she can try to discuss his situation as objectively as possible with her colleagues in the team at base. This seems to divert Jenny away from attacking Jon.

Nicola is realising that Jon will probably need to be on his own before an accurate assessment can be obtained. Subjectively she feels that he has an aura of depression about him. He looks defeated by his situation, although as yet it remains unclear what 'the situation' is. He appears to be the focus of blame by his wife. Nicola wonders how much of this is a 'projection' (Stuart and Laraia 2001) on Jenny's part to try to obliterate or divert from her own role in this relationship.

At the team assessment meeting it is agreed that he needs help, and that the team is the appropriate medium for this. Nicola is happy to take Jon on to her caseload. She sends him a letter asking him to attend a meeting at her base, where she hopes he will be able to speak more freely without his wife being there. Nicola and Jon have their first meeting at base, without Jenny being present:

Nicola. Hi, Jon, thanks for coming. Tell me what's been happening.

She notices immediately how much worse he looks. He is having difficulty maintaining any eye contact at all with her. He looks dishevelled. Nicola decides to address a vital area, the risk to Jon.

Her tone of voice is gentle, firm, concerned. She asks directly for what she needs to know. She uses a closed question but she feels that at the moment this is appropriate. It is important that she accurately assesses the depth of Jon's potential suicide intent before they part. (A way of assessing this might be to use a tool such as the Beck Depression Inventory.) She is able to use closed questions because with her he is not defensive. He is starting to let her help. There could be several reasons for this. He is certainly less resistant and evasive than when he was initially talking with Dr Stevens.

Discussion point

What do you think the reasons for this could be?

Jon. I found that difficult – indicating that I'd thought about ending my life. Jenny would kill me if she knew.

He laughs at the irony of this, and then suddenly looks as if he is going to burst into tears.

> Nicola. How was that difficult for you, Jon?

Again you can see that Nicola's deliberate use of questioning style retains the focus of the session, which is to accurately assess Jon's level of intention to carry out any thoughts of self-harm. She also, however, leaves plenty of space for Jon to express how he is feeling and what he is thinking. The balance here is heavily weighted towards Jon. Nicola is doing most of the listening, Jon is doing most of the talking. By the end of this first session of implementing the planned care as a result of the initial assessment, Nicola is reassured that Jon is often thinking of his own death but will not carry out any action to end his life because of his love for his sons and his perception of the impact this act would have on them. He does not seem to include Jenny in this particular concern.

As well as assessing in more depth this aspect of Jon's situation Nicola also makes an opportunity towards the end of the session to re-address the topic of Jon's view of his prescribed medication:

> Nicola. We need to talk about taking antidepressants again, Jon. It's important that you try them, as well as the work we're doing in these sessions. We stand a better chance of helping you if you'll give them a go. What do you think?
> Jon. OK. I'm not happy about taking them, but I'll give them a try. Would I be able have something else? Those others didn't seem to do anything for me.
> Nicola. Why don't you talk to Dr Stevens again and see what he thinks?

The evidence from a long history of research indicates that the combination of medication and use of psychosocial interventions seems to be helpful for people with depression (Newell and Gournay 2000). This is why Nicola is introducing the idea of Jon taking antidepressants again. She directs Jon back to his GP to maintain and promote the feeling for Jon that he has some say in what is happening to him. She is aware of how easily people can become disempowered when they become 'clients'.

During the third session Nicola starts to see evidence of some other issues that have as yet only been hinted at:

> Nicola. Tell me about the antidepressants? Any changes for the better yet?
> Jon. Nothing yet. Seeing you seems to help for a bit, but then after a day or two I feel just as bad. Just being able to say things without someone jumping down my throat is good.
> Nicola. What do you mean, 'jumping down my throat?' (repeating back the imagery used by Jon)
> Jon. I mean at home when I try to explain to Jenny what's going on, she gets really nasty. I've given up. We hardly speak. She's started to sleep in the spare room now. We try to hide it from the boys, but they know.
> Nicola. What do think is behind her nastiness towards you?

Nicola again has used the same language as Jon. She is focusing in on this aspect of Jon's story. Jon starts to explain some of the history of their relationship. It seems that the tension between them has been going on for several years. Jon tells Nicola that he had an affair at work with a colleague. It only lasted a few weeks but things have never been the same. Jon and Jenny don't talk about it. It is clear that Jon's story is becoming more and more convoluted. He is addressing things that appear to have been hidden for a long time. Nicola helps Jon tell his story by using basic interpersonal skills focused around a small cluster of intentions. Her intentions are to:

- Encourage Jon to tell his story (see also Egan stage 1 in Appendix B)
- Help him reveal how he feels about this
- Support him as he is doing this.

This is possibly the first time Jon has ever revealed this much of the story and the secrets he has been carrying around in his head for years. He even surprises himself sometimes as he feels safer and safer to say what is *really* on his mind but that he has never dared to say. He feels absolutely accepted by Nicola. It's as if he can say anything he wants to.

Together with these three basic intentions, Nicola's role is to monitor his mood to ensure he is safe (from himself). She then needs to make sure that he is being compliant as regards his medication, otherwise it is impossible to measure the effectiveness of the antidepressants. Next in the hierarchy of intentions is to facilitate the catharsis of thoughts, feelings and ideas that Jon seems to have suppressed for a long time. This is guided by him and not forced by her:

> **Jon.** Do you mind me talking about all this stuff? I thought you were meeting me to help me with my so called depression?
> **Nicola.** It sounds as if you're more angry than depressed at this moment
> **Jon.** Yes I bloody do feel angry, really angry. . . .

After about an hour of Jon revealing a range of things from his marriage, his work and his childhood, Nicola is aware that the session must come to a close. This is a skill that is needed whether you are working in a community setting or an institutional setting. Often there are pressures on you to be doing other things during your working day, as well as seeing individual clients. You have to find the way to 'wind down' an interaction to some kind of natural conclusion for the person in front of you. The sense is that of finishing the chapter for today, to be continued tomorrow, or next week, or next month, whenever your next meeting is.

Eventually, a session finish will be the last one, and that is something that you should prepare the person for from the very first meeting (section 2.22). Nicola brought this subject up with Jon when she made the first telephone contact. She said that they would meet for 6 weeks at first to see how things went, and then re-assess whether or not any more would be useful for Jon. This is one way of indicating the boundaries of the relationship.

Summary of skills used

- A rapport is started very quickly. There are always going to be difficulties around this in a community setting because the intervention opportunities are more limited than in institutional settings.
- A great deal of time is spent by Nicola in listening and encouraging Jon to talk. She uses open questioning to achieve this.
- Nicola uses her intuition. She sometimes has a 'hunch' about things and she uses this to develop the stage of care she is working through. (Egan, 2002,

talks about the idea of using hunches in connection with the concept of advanced empathy. Some professionals use this skill more than others.)

- She is very clear what her intentions are, although they are likely to change as her relationship with Jon changes. She also retains the flexibility to change her intention if it seems to be inappropriate.
- The use of silence and space is particularly important in this relationship. Jon seems to have many issues 'bottled up'.
- Jon's own language and imagery is used by Nicola to encourage him to expand on the statements he makes.
- She is sensitive to the timing of her visits. They are spaced to allow time for reflection and processing by Jon.
- The ending of the professional relationship is signalled at the start of it, probably the first meeting after the initial assessment. Nicola makes it clear that there is a clear number to the meetings they have. A review is held at that point to decide if they carry on, if Jon is to be referred elsewhere (perhaps back to his GP), or if he no longer needs input from the team member.

Summary of approaches used to make up strategy

Throughout their meetings Nicola uses a person-centred (or humanistic/ Rogerian) approach. She encourages Jon to tell his story, which relates to Egan's first stage of the helping process (see Appendix B). She is clear all the way through what her intentions are. She is very supportive, sometimes prescriptive, occasionally cathartic (Heron). She is aware that antidepressants can sometimes help so she uses a medical model approach in that sense. She liaises with the GP and her colleagues at base and in this way works collaboratively, although this is probably not apparent to Jon.

Prognosis

It looks from the dialogue above that the time for Nicola's interventions may be reaching the a natural conclusion, or at least a point where a review will be necessary. It could be that Jon is reaching a point where Nicola has helped him to access material that needs longer-term help and expertise, but not by a mental health specialist. A more appropriate person to help Jon, on a this type of basis, might be someone like a GP-based practice counsellor.

Jon carries on his meetings with the practice counsellor for a few weeks. In turn she suggests that Jon and Jenny seek help from Relate. Jon is reasonably happy with this as he feels it is a continuation of what he has already been doing. Jenny is unwilling at first but eventually agrees to see if it will help. Jon continues to take the antidepressants that Dr Stevens prescribed. He never is sure if the medication did anything. He insists that 'the talking seems to help most'.

5.5 LONG-TERM/CHRONIC PSYCHOSIS – LAURA

Preamble

It can be difficult to tell psychosis from depression in some people until a period of time has elapsed and you have got to know the person better.

The signs and symptoms that are similar to those of depression are known as 'negative symptoms' (Charlton 2000). These can cause the person to appear to be socially shy, withdrawn, lethargic, apathetic, apparently lacking in any desire to be socially integrated. It is only when you have gone further into the assessment process that you realise that the person is not only socially disadvantaged by the above but may well also be inappropriate in the way they express ideas. You may find that their way of looking at the world is unusual to say the least. They may be affected by delusional thinking, paranoia, or hallucinations (Wright and Giddey 1993). The person who suffers from these 'positive symptoms' is less likely to be mistakenly diagnosed as being depressed. The subject of the following story, Laura, seems to be suffering from a cluster of symptoms that would, at the moment, probably be recognised as 'positive symptons'.

Profile

Laura is a 29-year-old single woman. She frequently starts to sleep rough in her neighbourhood, despite having a flat. She pays the rent sporadically. Some of her fellow tenants express their concern to the landlord. He informs the police, out of concern for her rather than vindictiveness. The policewoman who speaks to Laura suggests that she sees her GP as soon as possible. The landlord's wife says she'll take her to the surgery.

Laura presents at the GP's surgery in a distracted and preoccupied state. The GP feels that Laura should be assessed at the local acute psychiatric unit. He is worried for her safety because of her increasing tendency to sleep outside – and the landlord reports that her flat is 'in a real mess'. After much persuasion from the landlord's wife, Laura agrees to be taken to the unit. On the drive there, Laura constantly looks around her. She says that she thinks they are 'being followed', and she seems to be in a state of hypervigilance.

Pathway through a long-term chronic psychosis

Laura is met at the ward front door by Dave, an experienced staff nurse:

Dave. Come in, Laura, and have a seat. Do you want a drink while we're carrying out the assessment?

This is a greeting that combines everyday ordinariness and the widely recognised welcoming gesture of a drink. Dave's intention is to help Laura feel comfortable during what is likely to be a very uncomfortable time for her. Dave uses direct eye contact, smiles, and offers a handshake while he is saying this.

Dave may, however, have tried to introduce the idea of the assessment too quickly. Sometimes, as nurses, we don't appreciate what it must be like to be admitted to a unit like this. It is our territory and we are familiar with what goes on and the environment and faces around us. Does Laura actually understand why she is at the unit and what is going to happen? A better way might have been for Dave to explain the whole process first and make sure that Laura understands what is going to happen to her. Many patients are very unhappy at being in a mental health unit. They are understandably sometimes very resistant to what carers are trying to do. The first few minutes of any admission procedure can help to set the tone for the rest of that person's time in care.

Laura. No, thanks, I can't stop long. What if they find out where I am?

Dave has some difficulty explaining to Laura why she has been brought to the unit, but he manages to get through to her with gentle persistence. She is still very fidgety and eager to go. He needs to get on with the admission procedure but puts that on hold for a time. His priority here is to respond constructively to Laura's fears.

His intention throughout this delicate initial stage of the admission is to carefully engage Laura in the start of a relationship that she will find helpful, comfortable and supportive. He does this by asking open but quite focused questions. For example the following question is a direct response to Laura's expressed anxieties. It combines the characteristics of attempting not to reinforce Laura's suspicions but at the same time not disregard them as fantasy either. They may, after all, be true. It also checks out the reasons that Laura seems to be so afraid.

Dave. Could you tell me a bit more about these people that you think are following you? What do you think will happen to you?
Laura. (*Looks very preoccupied*) I don't know. They'll probably stab me or something. I think they were following us down here, but we gave them the slip.
Dave. So you'll be safe here? Have a drink. There's few things I need to check with you and then I'll show you around the unit and where you'll be staying for a bit.

Dave is steering the conversation back to the admission. Laura is not ready yet. She will need some more persuasion.

Laura. I'm not staying. They'll find me and stab me. I don't want to be here.
Dave. I'm going to stay with you to make sure you're OK, until we've finished sorting out these details. After that, Ayesha (*a health-care assistant*) will be with you. We'll make sure someone is with you, or very near by. See how that is for you.

Again, Dave is here putting the administrative part of the admission on hold. His first priority is to try to reassure Laura in realistic way – i.e. a way that means something *to Laura*.

Laura is worried about her personal safety. She feels this is out of control. Dave is saying things that can be actually carried out and made real to Laura. He is not offering false promises that will erode the relationship rather than consolidate it. When she sees that what Dave says becomes reality, Dave has taken another step towards a relationship of trust that will be a key factor in Laura's recovery.

Laura. Why don't you just let me go home?
Dave. Well your landlord and friends and neighbours have been worried about you. Jane brought you down here didn't she, as she was so concerned?

Here Dave is reinforcing the reasons why Laura has been brought to the unit. He is trying to avoid the situation that often happens, when people are detained under a section of the Mental Health Act. He is trying to maintain Laura's current status as an informal admission. The very process of sectioning people often represents a serious setback to the formation of the helping relationship. It can alienate patients and make the job of helping them back to mental health so much more difficult. In effect it gives the patient yet another problem that they didn't have before being given the status of 'patient'.

It seems, from the subsequent conversation during the initial assessment and following admission, that Laura has lost contact with all her family, apart from her father, with whom she has a strained relationship. He reports that she sometimes becomes very aggressive towards him. She is in almost constant fear of being pursued by 'strangers'. At this point in her story with Dave, she is very vague. She returns again to the subject of people following her:

> **Laura.** Anyway, I don't want to talk any more. I need to get going before they trace me.
> **Dave.** Tell me again, who do you think is looking for you?
> **Laura.** Those *strangers*!
> **Dave.** What are they like?
> **Laura.** They scare me. I don't want to talk about them. You wouldn't understand anyway.

At this point Laura is giving away little pieces of information to Dave, from whom she may be feeling a lot of pressure. She gives away as little as possible. Why should she anyway, she hardly knows him, and what does *he* know?

She has a point here. She doesn't know anything about Dave as a person and doesn't want to. She has had very mixed experiences of psychiatric nurses and doctors in the past. In her view, some are OK, they seem quite kind, but some are 'bastards' and just want to keep you in hospital for as long as they can. Why does Dave want to know all this stuff about her? He'll probably end up using it against her anyway. He doesn't believe that she's being followed. He hasn't a clue how it is for her.

> **Dave.** We'll make sure that you're safe here. This will mean that some of the nurses will be keeping an eye on you until you settle in. Do you understand why we are doing this?
> **Laura.** No not really. I want to go.

Dave is having to be very persistent and patient. Laura keeps bringing up the same issues with dogged determination. In *her* world, someone is following her, she doesn't want to be in hospital and this nurse is pressuring her to stay by making all sorts of promises. She's heard it all before.

Despite all this initial difficulty, Dave does eventually manage to persuade Laura to stay, with the help of Rose. Rose is a retired nursing officer doing the occasional bank nurse shift, and remembers Laura from 10 years ago. Laura remembers her also. Laura remembers Rose's kindness as much as anything else. Rose plays a large part in persuading Laura to stay on the ward.

They suggest that Laura tries to stay until the weekend and sees how she feels then. Dave knows that the chances of her being sectioned under the Mental Health Act are quite high if she tries to go. It is likely that any doctor who assessed her would see her as being potentially unsafe. At this stage Dave has tried to obtain some insight into how Laura is seeing her situation. He has attempted to assess the robustness of her delusions (he would need to confirm that they are delusions). She needs some time to settle down and get used to the new people around her. He tries to re-explain why she will be under observation and attempts to confirm her understanding of this.

> Dave. Laura, while you're here I'm going to arrange for someone to be with you or near you as I said earlier. This is so that we can make sure you're OK and safe all the time you are here. Please don't think that we are following you. I'll be with you some of the time, so will Rose. At other times some of the other nurses will be with or near you.

Laura seems to understand this. Over the next few days there is the first evidence that she is starting to mellow a little in her hostility and resistance. She has started to accept small doses of an antipsychotic drug that she agrees to take from Rose. Whether or not the changes in her are anything to do with this remains unclear. Nevertheless, the care team keep up their strategy of gentle persistence in monitoring Laura. They are making sure she is safe, and consolidating and gradually building the depth and quality of the relationship she has, not just with Dave and Rose but with all members of the care team.

A few days later...

> Dave. How are you getting on?

Dave is aware that Laura has been very restless during the night and on a couple of occasions has demanded to go home in the early hours. The night staff have managed to persuade her otherwise. They have done this by again maintaining a strategy of gentle, persistent persuasion. This is where the investment that the nursing staff have made in the relationship they have with Laura pays off. A confrontation is avoided and Laura acquiesces.

> Laura. I'm fine, thanks.

Her affect is flat when she says this and she gives Dave no eye contact. Her response is incongruent. What she is saying doesn't seem to ring true. Dave gently picks up on this.

> Dave. You don't really look 'fine'. I understand that you've not been sleeping very well lately?

Dave's intention here is to work a little on trying to get some depth into the assessment of how Laura is. He does this by challenging or confronting Laura but in a very low key way. This is another test of just how trusting the relationship has become.

> Laura. Who told you that?
> Dave. Joan, the nurse who was on duty last night, said you were restless and up and about several times. What's happening?
> Laura. I keep waking up and thinking they're in the room with me. Joan makes me think it's all right. She makes me feel better. I can get off to sleep but then it happens again. So I get up and go and see her again.
> Dave. Good. That's OK. You must keep doing that. Joan is good isn't she?

Here Dave is trying to work therapeutically at several different levels:

- He does not try to persuade Laura that the people in her room don't exist
- He supports and validates Laura's way of managing this difficult situation for herself
- He supports his colleague, Joan, in what she is doing
- He is openly and realistically optimistic and positive
- He validates Joan's actions. In doing this he is slowly increasing the size of the support network that Laura feels comfortable with
- He is at the same time reducing her dependence on a small number of carers and dissipating it around more people
- He is helping her work out for herself what managing strategies work for her
- He is gradually helping her re-build her sense of self-esteem
- He is gently becoming engaged in the more complex problems that Laura is experiencing.

Laura is still very suspicious and resistant. She will need a gentle approach before she starts to tell the nursing staff how she really feels. This could take weeks. It may not happen at all. The strategy the care team have is to keep chipping away through her defences. It is important to realise that her defences are probably based on fear. To her the threat from the strangers is real. How does she know for sure that the care team are not in league with the strangers? It can be, of course, difficult to empathise with someone whose truth is so distorted and distant from the reality that most of us function in, most of the time. Dave has a go.

> **Dave.** Hi, Laura. How's it going today for you?
> **Laura.** The strangers haven't tried to get on to the ward yet. I wish they'd just leave me alone
> **Dave.** It must be really horrible for you, this feeling that the strangers could come at any time?
> **Laura.** Yes, it is horrible.

At this moment Laura, for the first time, gives Dave direct and steady eye contact. She has found someone who really seems to understand what it is like for her. At this same instant Dave realises that he has made an important break-through. They have connected.

The significance of this interaction should not be underestimated. The technique that Dave attempted was an empathic intervention. He was trying to capture the sense of what Laura must be experiencing, and he tried to communicate that back to her. This style of intervention is very helpful, when it works, in terms of its ability to deepen the relationship. Even if it doesn't work, the technique can still contribute to the data that Dave is acquiring each occasion he spends time with Laura. This is how it might have gone, if Dave had not been so accurately empathic:

> **Dave.** It must be really horrible for you, this feeling that the strangers could come at any time?
> **Laura.** It's not horrible – it's making me tired and angry. I'm worn out – I wish they'd leave me alone.

Dave has not been on target with his empathic attempt but it has still helped

Laura reveals a little more about how she feels and how it is affecting her. The point here is that, whether or not the empathic intervention works, it still is beneficial to make the thoughtful attempt.

From now on, Laura feels she has something of an ally. A possibility is that she may be increasingly likely to tell Dave how her world is. His skilled responses to this world can be tremendously important in Laura's recovery.

Part of Dave's bigger role is to be constantly attempting to realistically reassure Laura that other members of the care team will be able to listen to her and help her as well. He does this earlier by encouraging the relationships with Rose and Joan, two colleagues for whom Laura feels some connection. Otherwise the responsibility for Dave can become very onerous. The professional relationship between Dave and Laura can start to work on a higher level.

> **Dave.** How's your day been? Did you go with Ayesha to visit your flat?
> **Laura.** It was good. The flat was a bit musty so we let some fresh air through it. The strangers weren't waiting for me. I checked while Ayesha was there.
> **Dave.** What did Ayesha say about the strangers?
> **Laura.** She said not to worry about them as they weren't real, even though I think they are. She said to think how many times I'd actually seen them for myself. My dad always used to ignore me when I talked about them, or he'd laugh at me.
> **Dave.** Perhaps your dad didn't know how to handle your ideas. Maybe he was concerned but couldn't show it. That must have hurt, that he seemed to ignore what you said.
> **Laura.** Whatever. He was never much use anyway. At least Ayesha seems to try.
> **Dave.** Anyway, you could go to the flat again tomorrow with Ayesha and have another look. See what you think.

There is some evidence that there may be some unresolved issues around the relationship that Laura has with her father. Dave mentally notes this, and later he will make an entry in her care plan that this might be an area that could be addressed at some time in the future, if it ever becomes appropriate. In the meantime he is dealing, in a practical way, with getting Laura back to her flat.

At the same time Dave is still not totally denying the existence of the strangers. He is relying on Laura to again work through a process herself with the support of another trusted carer, Ayesha. This is a Socratic process. Laura will work out reality herself, and Dave is trying to give her the space to do this. At the same time, the team is making sure that she is safe and complying with other structured care such as the administration of any medication.

Note that throughout this process Laura's mood seems to mellow. Her responses to caring interventions become more reasoned and less reactive and suspicious. It is noticeable that, when Laura is first assessed and admitted, her personality seems cold and hard-edged. This can be typical of people who suffer from long term psychotic difficulties. Their personality in times of relapse seems colder, more distant and less willing to engage with others than in times of remission. Now Laura shows signs of warmth, sometimes, to members of the ward team that she knows well and feels familiar with. She seems softer and more spontaneous in her interactions, although she still has to be approached and won't usually start a conversation first. This could of course be her premorbid personality, i.e. her usual healthy personality.

Laura has very little to do to with the other patients on the ward at the moment. In that sense, the process of developing a therapeutic relationship consisting of acceptance, respect, genuineness and trust is very little different from the process with any other type of patient. Fortunately her progress like this continues gradually. She starts going out to stay overnight at her flat.

The community mental health team take her on to their caseload. Things are going well for her over the next few months. Then, when her community psychiatric nurse calls, on several occasions she is out. The CPN leaves several notes asking Laura to call. She doesn't respond to any of these. The CPN, during the first of these visits, was accompanied by student nurse Sharon Green. It is a continuation of Sharon's branch community placement. She seemed to get on OK with Laura. Sharon felt quite pleased with herself. CPN Ruth Simpson suggests to Sharon that every other visit she sees Laura on her own. Laura was asked about this and seemed fine with the idea. She was happy to help a student.

Then Laura 'disappears'. This has a surprising effect on Sharon. She feels let down by Laura. She wonders about her own professional ability to create trusting relationships and her ability to judge how patients are going to react. She thought, when Laura said she'd see her in a couple of weeks' time to have her regular depot injection and a chat, that she really meant it.

Ruth feels the need to try to reassure Sharon. She is used to this kind of situation. It's just the nature of the job. This is how people are sometimes, not just in mental health nursing. Many people aren't totally reliable. Just think how many times you've been let down by people outside of working as a mental health nurse. Mental illness probably just exaggerates a little what is already there. This is the first time that Sharon has felt this way, but it won't be the last. The things that Ruth says to her are written down by Sharon in her reflective portfolio as an 'informal' supervision session. It seems to help her.

> Sharon. It feels like it's almost my fault that Laura's disappeared again. I didn't pick up that anything was wrong. She seemed OK, didn't she? I wonder how I'm ever going to really get to grips with this client group?
> Ruth. This situation is very common. People like Laura are very difficult to keep engaged. Sometimes that's because of their natural personality, sometimes it's the illness, sometimes it's a combination of both. When you work with this group of people you have to get used to this. Probably, at the time you saw her, she did intend to meet for her medication and to have your chat. It's difficult to tell whether this is absent-mindedness because she's preoccupied, or deliberate resistance and avoidance. Whatever, we need to keep trying to make contact. How about you write to her asking her to phone us at base, and I'll call in tomorrow to see if she's around. I'm going past her flat anyway.

Sharon appreciates Ruth's help, but she is still not convinced. How could she have misread that situation so badly? When she was working with Joanne as a client, things seemed much clearer. All the time she went to see Joanne (see 5.3) at her home, she thought she had a good sense of what therapeutic relationships were. She could see her own relationship-building skills developing as well. Now she feels de skilled, almost as if she's learned nothing.

Ruth continues to support Sharon while she gets her confidence back. She is keen to help Sharon see that Laura's absence is not a personal rebuttal. It is a natural part of mental health nursing and caring. It might even be seen as some patients and clients 'testing' their carers. Some people who suffer from mental illness have been let down by significant others in their relationships. Why shouldn't others do the same to them? Given how staff and students move around and are transient, for many different reasons, it is not difficult to understand the reticence of patients and clients to trust in the longevity of our relationships with them.

A few weeks later, Laura is readmitted to the ward. It appears that she has been sleeping rough just outside the grounds of the local general hospital for several days. She is brought into the mental health unit by the police, who recognise her. She has lost a lot of weight, looks bedraggled and again is scared of 'them following me'. That is the reason she gives for sleeping rough. 'They' know where she lives, and this is the only way to escape. She is admitted to the same ward that she was on several weeks ago. Her new named nurse is struggling with her. Dave is not back on duty until tomorrow.

> **Carol.** Hi, Laura I'm your named nurse while you're here. Could we talk for a few minutes. I wasn't here when you were admitted last time.
> **Laura.** I want to go. They know I'm here.
> **Carol.** We can't let you go at the moment. The police have brought you in because people are worried about you again, Laura.

Carol tries to use the persuasive argument that last time Laura was in she didn't have to stay long. Nothing awful happened to her and she was quickly able to return home. Contemporary practice suggests that, if relapsing clients can be treated early enough by intervening when their prodromal symptoms become apparent, then their stay in hospital (if necessary) is likely to be shorter. They may not even need admission at all. Prodromal symptoms are the signs and symptoms that signal the possible start of relapse: 'They are unique to each person and are also known as the relapse signature' (O'Brien *et al.* 1999, p. 288).

This is a very delicate situation for Carol. Again, Laura is on the cusp of leaving the ward and similarly Carol is on the edge of applying a nurse's holding power (Section 5.4 of the Mental Health Act 1983) if Laura insists on going. She has tried contacting the duty doctor to visit urgently, but the doctor is not available.

And so the conversation goes on. It is similar in content to the last time that Laura was in hospital. Despite this, the work of the nursing staff is no easier, especially the ones who have not met Laura before. They seemingly have to build the rapport up from nothing. This is very hard and tiring work. But it's different for Dave, who returns the next day.

> **Dave.** Hi, Laura. Back with us again for a while? It won't be long, with a bit of luck, will it?
> **Laura.** I want to go. Please let me out. You know I hate it in here.
> **Dave.** I seem to remember that last time you were here, we went on that trip to the cinema with Joan and the others. Do you remember? And what about when we watched that programme on TV together? I've never seen you laugh so much!

Laura. I know, I was OK then. They stopped following me.
Dave. So maybe the same will happen again if you stick with it for a bit?

Here Dave is using his previous effective relationship with Laura for an immediately useful purpose. His intention is to try to remind Laura of the positive memories that she might have about being in hospital on this ward and the special nature of the relationship that she and Dave have developed. Even though patients leave the ward or are discharged from your case load, the work you have invested into the relationship is often still there dormant, waiting to be rekindled for the benefit of the patient, if and when you meet again. Your colleagues can sometimes usefully tap into this resource.

Laura's stay this time is not quite as long as the last time. The care team seem to have found a combination of intervention styles, activities and medication that speeds the process of helping her return to health. The relationships she has with Dave, Rose, Joan and now Carol help to facilitate this. She is discharged back to her flat with the same package of after care. Again, Ruth picks up her case. Five months later she is admitted again.

Summary of skills used

- Dave has a persona of being 'ordinary.' This helps to make him a little more approachable to Laura who at the moment will regard most people with a degree of suspicion.
- His intention at the start of the relationship is to try to create a rapport. Again, this is very difficult with people suffering with this kind of suspicious or paranoid mindset.
- Right from the start, Dave creatively tries to empower Laura by offering her as much choice as the immediate situation allows. He is trying to maintain what little sense of control she has in an out of control situation (for her).
- He is gently persistent. He will need to be, as Laura is very resistant at the moment. How much of this is because of her premorbid personality (her natural, healthy personality) and how much because of her illness is, at the time of admission, unclear.
- He uses open questioning techniques but sometimes tempered with a closed approach, as appropriate.
- Sometimes it seems more helpful to Laura for Dave and the team to be rather more directive with her. There is of course a tension here between the way we are directive towards patients in institutional settings, and the need to empower.
- Dave is clear about his intentions. Some of these in the early stages of the admission would be to:
  - Gain information and encourage insight – catalytic
  - See how she feels – cathartic
  - Tell her what is happening – informative
- He is honest with Laura, even if this brings short-term difficulties. She may not like what she is hearing: 'The doctor has prescribed this medication for you'. Dave's honesty is more likely to bring longer-term benefits for Laura, as she wants to know what is happening to her. Any inconsistency from the care team may only serve to reinforce her suspicions.
- Dave uses his intuition. He sometimes senses what Laura is feeling or is about to do.

- He tries to be empathic. This is to signal to Laura that he is trying to understand how things are for her. To attempt this with any patient or client often has great value.
- Dave is consistently supportive. He is aware of the difficulty that might arise when the team needs to restrict her movements if she becomes a formal patient (detained under the Mental Health Act). Her view of him may flip from seeing him as a carer to seeing him as a form of policeman.

Summary of approaches used to make up strategy

The care team work collaboratively. Dave uses a person-centred approach. He is accepting and empathic. He constantly tries to empower Laura in an institutional setting that is naturally disempowering. He is clear about his intentions. He is sometimes prescriptive, sometimes catalytic, sometimes cathartic. He uses a gently challenging approach to help Laura question the reality of her delusions, whenever appropriate.

Prognosis

Laura's future is likely to be a pattern of remission and relapse that Laura may have to endure. Historically it has been suggested that around a third of people who suffer from schizophrenia experience this type of cycle (Newell and Gournay 2000). Often, it seems that stress may trigger off relapse (Gelder *et al.* 1999). Also, it is thought that if the sufferer is part of a highly critical family dynamic (high expressed emotion – HEE), then the likelihood of relapse is increased (O'Brien *et al.* 1999). There is some evidence that, if sufferers are able to keep in contact with an effective support worker using a contemporary approach such as an educative/supportive role with the family as well as the carer, the prognosis is improved (Gelder *et al.* 1999).

5.6 ACUTE PSYCHOSIS – WENDY

Preamble

Acute psychosis is often much easier to spot during clinical assessment as the signs and symptoms are much clearer. The sufferer may be irritated and worried, or tormented and frightened, by existing in a world that many of us only experience when we have nightmares (Barry 1998, Gelder *et al.* 1999). Sufferers from active psychosis may think that they are being followed, that others are out to get them. They may hear voices that insult them and belittle them or, most worryingly, voices that tell them to do things (command hallucinations, see Varcarolis 1998).

As with the more long-term psychosis described in the previous section, a contemporary approach is to try to engage with the sufferer and their family. If this is achieved then there is more chance that the sufferer's prodromal symptoms or relapse signature can be recognised. Action can then be taken to try to avoid a full slip into relapse. Alternatively, the relapse can sometimes be better managed by altering the medication to find a new therapeutic level. Another option is finding a more effective medication, together with a supportive interpersonal approach with the patient and their family.

Profile

Wendy is 19 years old. She is the youngest of three sisters. She studied away from home at a large university but had to return home after three semesters for 'time out'. Her fellow students and tutors were very worried about her behaviour. In class and socially she became very withdrawn. At night she could be heard having long conversations with people who, it transpired, were products of what looked like a psychosis.

Wendy's mother said that, looking back, this had been building up for about five years. The first signs started shortly after Wendy's father left the family when she was 14. At this stage she became withdrawn, but her mother attributed this to a period of bullying at school that she encountered. During this time Wendy's mother started to work again in paid employment after many years as a housewife. She returned to her former job as an outreach worker. This in turn seemed to trigger off some difficulties with Wendy's siblings. There were many arguments in the house. Recently, Wendy has been going out in the early hours of the morning to get away from the people in her room. After a home visit, the family's GP is concerned enough to arrange assessment at the local acute psychiatric unit.

Pathway through acute psychosis

Wendy has recently been admitted to an acute psychiatric unit. On admission she was surprisingly aggressive for such a normally quiet personality:

> **Sylvia.** Wendy, welcome to the unit. We'll show you around in a few minutes. I just need to ask you a few questions first.
> **Wendy.** You can get lost, I'm not talking to anyone.
> **Sylvia.** OK. We'll leave it for a bit. Have a seat. I'll nip and get you a drink first. Tea, coffee or fruit juice?
> **Wendy** (*mumbles*). Coffee, no sugar.

This difficult exchange is significant for several reasons:

- Sylvia is being consistently warm and welcoming. She is like this regardless of the mental state of any patient.
- She is informing. She tells Wendy what is happening and what is going to happen. This is her intention.
- Wendy is resistant and un-co-operative. She may be frightened, angry, confused, embarrassed.
- The nurse acquiesces with what Wendy wants as much as she can. There is no point in getting locked into an exchange of 'Yes, you will' – 'No, I won't' at any stage of the admission, although sometimes this is very difficult to avoid.
- The nurse's acquiescence achieves the first little bit of evidence that Wendy may be willing to at least listen. This is a significant advance and has been achieved within two nursing interventions.
- The nurse gives Wendy some space now while she makes a drink. It would be very prudent to ensure that Wendy is observed discreetly by another experienced member of staff to monitor the situation.

> **Sylvia.** Here's your coffee, Wendy (*waits for her to take a few sips*). So what's been happening at home? I understand you've not been getting much sleep?

Here Sylvia is intention-driven again. Her intentions are:

- To reassure and support
- To try to further develop the rapport that is attempted through the giving of the drink
- To obtain pieces of information that are easy and non-threatening for Wendy to talk about.
- To do this in a way that is very open at first – 'What's been happening at home?' Then becoming a little more focused – 'I understand you've not been getting much sleep?' There is some safety built into this for Wendy, as she has the choice which of these she wishes to answer, the general question or the specific question.

Sylvia has exerted a little bit of subtle pressure on Wendy by giving her a choice of two questions to respond to rather than a choice of responding to one question or not responding at all. It's rather like the salesman's closing question of 'Do you want the car in blue or red?'

There is a high level of skill involved at this stage of admitting and assessing a difficult/resistant/non-compliant person into an institutional setting. The nurse needs to be welcoming but professional, relaxed but business-like, in control but empowering. These skills are most desirable at this very important stage in the person's process through the illness. They can set the tone for the rest of the person's experience in that care setting.

Wendy is persuaded to stay, largely by the skills of Sylvia in creating a working rapport where at first there was coldness and resistance. Wendy agrees to take medication before Sylvia goes off duty:

> **Sylvia.** The doctor who came to see you earlier prescribed a sleeping tablet and a drug to start helping you with these strange thoughts.
> **Wendy.** What's that one called?
> **Sylvia.** The sleeping tablet is zopiclone and the other one is risperidone. It's a very small dose to see if it suits you. It's two a day. Would you be OK to take them? They usually help, in my experience. If you find they're not helping or they make you feel worse in some way, you can stop.
> **Wendy.** I'll try them for a few days, I suppose.

Over the next few days Wendy maintains an air of suspicion and withdrawal. It is not always clear that she has taken her medication. Some of the other patients complain about her to the staff. Wendy is found to have removed personal belongings from other patients' lockers. She is also keeping leftover food in her own locker. She remains unsociable and antisocial.

> **Sylvia.** Hi, Wendy. Could we have a few minutes together later on this morning? I'll come and get you in an hour. Is that OK?
> **Wendy** nods agreement but doesn't give Sylvia any eye contact.

An hour later Sylvia goes back to meet Wendy. She is nowhere to be seen. A colleague says that he thinks Wendy has gone to the shop for cigarettes. An hour later Wendy is seen sitting on her own in the smoking area of the ward.

> **Sylvia.** Hi, Wendy. I missed you earlier. I came to find you as we agreed but you were out. Shall we have some time now?

As always, Sylvia is directed by her intentions, which are to:

- Re-establish rapport by remaining consistently friendly, accepting, non-judgemental (on the surface anyway – sometimes we struggle with these issues)
- Inform Wendy what has happened
- Re-state their agreement, but not in any punitive sense
- Try to find out more about Wendy by creating opportunities whenever she can. This is not the time to be precious about time and contractual boundaries.

Sylvia spends some time with Wendy. Her intentions over this period are to:

- Invest further in the rapport they have
- Find out more about Wendy's history
- See how she is feeling
- See what she is thinking
- Report back to the team verbally, if she has any immediate concerns, and by using Wendy's care notes for longer term material.

Within a couple of weeks, the efforts of the care team, and Sylvia as Wendy's named nurse, seem to be having a positive effect. Wendy has been co-operative, on the whole, about taking her medication. Occasionally she has refused but that is usually because she has been offered it by a member of staff to whom she has taken an intense dislike. All they need to do to manage the situation is to ask someone else on the shift to administer Wendy's medication and that gets around the problem without making it more complex than it need be. What seems to be working with Wendy is the tried and tested combination of conservatively and thoughtfully applied medical model and creatively applied humanistic interventions.

It is Student Nurse Sharon Green's first day on the unit. It is her acute placement. Sylvia is her assessor. She introduces Sharon to Wendy. Wendy is very quiet and doesn't give Sharon much eye contact. She gives Sharon a limp and rather sweaty handshake. There is something about Wendy that Sharon really likes.

> **Sharon.** Nice to meet you, Wendy. Catch up with you later, perhaps?
> **Wendy.** Yeah. OK, maybe.

Sharon decides to go into the office to read Wendy's notes and care plan. She asks Sylvia if she could shadow her work with Wendy and be a supervised associate named nurse. Sylvia agrees as long as Sharon checks back with her what she's doing. Sharon reads all about Wendy's time at university and the struggles at home after her father left. This strikes a chord with Sharon. Her own father left the family when she was 10. She sees little of him to this day. Sharon sees Wendy sitting on her own looking out of the window. She has a plan. She will try to strike up a conversation with Wendy and gradually work it around to the relationship between Wendy and her father. It does say in the care plan that this might be an area to explore, if and when appropriate.

> **Sharon.** Hi, Wendy, do you mind if I sit with you for a bit?
> **Wendy.** Suit yourself.
> **Sharon.** How are you settling now? I understand from Sylvia that you've not been too keen to take your medication? Don't you find it helps you?

Wendy. The sleepers are OK, but the other one makes me feel weird sometimes. It's OK, I'll keep going. Sylvia says I seem better, and my mum agrees.

Sharon. That's good. How does your mum manage all this? I understand that your dad isn't around? It must be difficult for her – and you?

Wendy. Hang on. What's he got to do with all this?

Sharon. Sorry, I thought you might like to talk about him.

Wendy. Well I don't. I want to forget all about him. (*Looks extremely annoyed and starts to shake slightly.*)

Sharon. I'm really sorry. I'll leave you alone for a bit.

Sharon is getting flustered. She goes to find Sylvia to tell her what has happened. She hears a wailing noise from the other end of the ward. Wendy has quickly become very distraught. One of the staff nurses is offering her some medication to 'calm you down a bit'. Wendy accepts this. Sharon feels stupid and embarrassed. She wishes she had been a little less pushy and a little more sensitive.

An hour later things are calmer. Wendy is fast asleep on her bed. Sylvia finds Sharon, who seems rather preoccupied.

Sylvia. Could we have a talk about what happened with Wendy?

Sharon. I'm really sorry, I feel so stupid.

Sylvia. It happens sometimes. Just talk me through what went on.

Sylvia's intentions here are as follows:

- She will explain to Sharon that their conversation is informal supervision. There is no punitive intent.
- She will feed back to Sharon the positive parts of the event and the negative parts
- She will be supportive to Sharon and constructive in her comments
- She regards this as an opportunity, rather than a damage-limitation exercise
- She will turn it into a learning experience for Sharon and an opportunity to use the interaction to help add more depth to Wendy's care plan.

Sharon explains her approach.

Sharon. I wanted to talk to Wendy about her dad. It was in the care plan. I thought I could try to empathise with her. My dad left too.

Sylvia explains that there are several reasons that probably contributed to Wendy becoming upset:

- Sharon had not invested enough time in building a rapport. With some people this happens very quickly, possibly in a few minutes. With other people it can take weeks, months or maybe it doesn't happen at all. Once the rapport is established, the carer can then start to work at a slightly deeper level when the opportunity presents. The experienced creative carer can contribute to the opportunities being created. This accelerates the process of caring, but never faster than the patient/client can manage.
- It is possible that Wendy experienced Sharon's intervention as being pushy and intrusive

- Sharon was probably over-identifying with Wendy. In some ways Sharon's experience might have some similarities. In other ways it will be entirely different. It is not helpful to believe that because you have had a similar experience to someone your feelings about it will also be similar.
- Sharon had helpful intentions but the outcome is not what she had anticipated. The area that Sharon was hoping to explore with Wendy was likely to be difficult and was only going to be approached by one of the more experienced staff if appropriate. Sylvia stresses that all interventions should be discussed with her first.

Throughout their discussion Sylvia is supportive of Sharon. She was trying to be helpful, but it didn't go as planned, in many ways. Sharon still feels that she 'messed up', even though Sylvia has tried to be constructive.

The next day Sharon approaches Wendy again:

Sharon. Hi, Wendy. How are you? I'm sorry about all that fuss yesterday.
Wendy. It's OK. I was a bit over the top. I'm a bit funny about my dad, especially in here. I've got too much time to think about things.
Sharon. In what way?
Wendy. I think about the months after he went, and how he doesn't seem to want to see us, even now.
Sharon. That must be really hard for you?
Wendy. It's the hardest thing, really. . . (*She becomes tearful again*).

Sharon's heart sinks. Wendy is going to get upset again and she'll look like she's caused it, and Sylvia will talk to her again and she'll get a bad report from this ward.

Sharon sits with Wendy for a few minutes, hoping that none of the other staff notice that she is upset again.

Wendy. Thanks for listening to me. I feel a bit better now.
Sharon. That's OK. I'm making a drink – do you want one?
Wendy. That would be great.

Suddenly Sharon feels she's done something useful.

Wendy seems to be making good progress during her time in hospital. She is becoming gradually more animated. She is making more effort to talk to other people on the ward. Her mum visits regularly as her other commitments allow. Wendy goes home for a couple of days at a weekend. On her return her mother reports to Sylvia that she hasn't slept much and has become more agitated and withdrawn over the two days. Last night she thought she could hear Wendy talking to someone in her room. Sylvia spends some time with Wendy once her mum has gone:

Sylvia. So how was the weekend?
Wendy. Mum must have told you. Not brilliant.
Sylvia. So, tell me the bad things that happened.
Wendy. I started to feel cut off again. There's lots of people to talk to here. I like talking to Sharon. My sisters were out a lot with their friends. While I was in my room last night I saw those people again.
Sylvia. The ones in your mind.

Wendy. Yes but they weren't in my mind, they were in my room again.

Sylvia. Well that's what it seems like. How did you feel about them appearing to be in your room? You must have been really annoyed?

Wendy. Yes, I felt cross with them and cross with myself. I'm supposed to be getting better aren't I?

Sylvia. You are getting better in many ways. If you weren't better we wouldn't be having this conversation. You wouldn't be making friends here. You wouldn't be talking to Sharon.

Wendy. I suppose so.

Sylvia. Anyway, what did you do next?

Wendy. I started shouting at them to go away. I put my TV on to take my mind off them. I kept the TV on all night. I couldn't sleep much. They didn't come back, though.

Sylvia. Sounds like the changes and the stress of going home might have triggered this off. But you found a way of managing it didn't you? In a funny sort of way it's good that the people came back because it helped you find a way of getting rid of them. At least for a while. It might be that sometimes they will come back, especially at times of change or stress. Now you've found a way of sorting them out for a while. Tell me about some of the good things that happened over the weekend?

Wendy. I had a good chat to my sisters when they were there. It was nice to be in my own space again for a bit, and play some CDs. They tend to go missing here, don't they? I suppose, as you say, it was good that I managed to sort out the people in my room. It's left me really tired, though.

Sylvia. How about having a lie down for an hour?

Throughout this difficult interaction, Sylvia has several intentions:

- To support Wendy and validate her actions
- To demonstrate empathy – 'You must have been really annoyed'
- To concentrate on the positive aspects of a difficult time for Wendy (cognitive re-framing)
- Not to reinforce or deny the existence of the 'people'
- To check how Wendy feels about this
- To remain realistically optimistic about Wendy
- To be tangibly caring and concerned.

Wendy goes on a couple more weekend leaves. One Sunday night the staff phone her at home and ask if she will stay at home. They have had to use her bed for an emergency admission. Wendy's mum phones the ward the following day and says that Wendy is now refusing to go back to hospital as she's 'fine now'.

Wendy is sent an appointment to come into the ward for a meeting with her consultant. He is considering discharging her. She doesn't reply but her mum again contacts the consultant and says that Wendy is refusing to see him as 'they're all the same'. It is not clear what Wendy means by this. The consultant refers Wendy to the community team. The CPN Ruth Simpson calls round to see Wendy. Her mum lets her into the house.

Wendy's mum is quite tearful. She thinks that Wendy might be relapsing again. She recognises the same behaviours that she has seen before. Ruth recognises these behaviours as Wendy's relapse signature (Birchwood *et al.* 1992, cited in Newell and Gournay 2000). Wendy refuses to come out of her bedroom.

Two months later she is re-admitted on to the ward. The efforts of Ruth and her colleagues have not managed to maintain Wendy at home. Student Nurse Sharon Green is still on the ward but is now nearly at the end of her placement. She and Sylvia are both on duty when Wendy arrives on the ward. The consultant thought it best to request this. He is aware of the good rapport that the two nurses have developed with Wendy. He thinks that the arranged admission will be most comfortable for Wendy if nurses that she knows are there for her on her arrival:

> **Sylvia.** Hi, Wendy. Really sorry to see you back. We hope it won't be for long, though. Here's Sharon as well, although she's only here for another couple of weeks.

Sylvia is making it clear that Sharon is not going to be around for much longer. She is aware that Wendy could become attached to a friendly face only for it to disappear soon.

> **Sharon.** Have a seat, Wendy. I'll get you a drink. Is it coffee?

Wendy just nods but doesn't speak. Sharon is a little surprised. What has happened to the rapport they had a couple of months ago? She has learned by now not to take this personally, like she used to when she first started her nurse training course. Sylvia has explained to her in the past that people are often very inward looking when they are suffering from mental illness. They are not, therefore, overly concerned with the feelings of others, especially professional carers with whom they come into contact.

> **Sharon.** Wendy, how are you doing? It must be strange to be back?
> **Wendy.** Whatever.
> **Sharon.** I'll just show you where your room is, Wendy. Then I'll leave you to it for a while. Could we have a chat about what's been happening, after you've had something to eat?
> **Wendy.** Yes ... I suppose so (*She seems a little irritated*).

Sharon is trying to achieve several aims here, although with limited success:

- Open questions are used to give the person space to answer
- The patient is given a base. A personal area is all-important to try to promote a feeling of individuality in an institutional setting
- Sharon gives Wendy some space and doesn't push her too hard – she has learned from her mistake last time
- She offers Wendy something to eat – she remembers to be aware of the person's basic needs
- She tries to get tacit agreement to continue the dialogue later so that, when Sharon re-approaches her, Wendy has some expectation that this will happen.
- It is absolutely essential that, if Sharon suggests this, she carries it out, even if there is a high risk of non-co-operation from Wendy.

Later that day...

> **Sharon.** How are you settling in, Wendy? Did you have anything to eat? Is your Mum visiting later?
>
> **Wendy.** What's this, twenty questions?

Sharon realises she is doing it again.

> **Sharon.** Sorry, I was just concerned, really. I'm sad to see you back.
>
> **Wendy.** Not as sad as me
>
> **Sharon.** How's it happened, anyway?
>
> **Wendy.** I felt so much better. Things were going well. I started to go out again. I wrote to a couple of universities to see if I could get a place for next year. I stopped taking the medication. The people came back, only worse than before. They are nasty to me now. They call me horrible things. I tried what Ruth said but it doesn't work any more. I didn't want to see her anyway. I thought she'd make me come back into hospital (*She starts to cry again*).

Sharon doesn't say anything at all. She sits quietly with Wendy.

Three weeks later, Wendy recovers enough to go home again, with support from Ruth, the CPN.

Summary of skills used

- Sylvia is consistent and approachable throughout her time with Wendy. This is sometimes difficult, because Wendy is sometimes very hostile.
- She constantly works to sustain a positive rapport. As above, this has its problems because of Wendy's changing demeanour.
- Sylvia uses open questions to give Wendy space to reflect on her situation.
- She gently challenges Wendy's perception of some situations.
- Sylvia is clear about her intentions but retains the ability to be flexible about them, if need be.
- Micro stories are used to utilise Sylvia's experiences to validate what Wendy is feeling (see also section 3.1).
- Sylvia is always honest with Wendy, even if this is sometimes uncomfortable for both of them. Sylvia's discomfort comes from knowing she may have to say something to Wendy that could upset her. Wendy's discomfort comes from being told something she may not want to hear.
- She remains professionally non-judgemental and accepting of Wendy.
- She tells Wendy what is going on. Her intention is to be informative
- Sylvia is supportive of Wendy.
- She maintains an attitude of realistic and cautious optimism.

Summary of approaches to make up strategy

Sylvia and the team are person-centred. They are consistently, accepting, warm, and they attempt to be empathic. Sylvia is clear about her intentions. She is supportive, prescriptive, informative and challenging when appropriate. The team uses the family as a therapeutic resource. The physical side of Wendy's care is considered in terms of hydration, nutrition, personal space, monitoring medication and so on.

Prognosis

The key issue here is likely to be the recognition of Wendy's prodromal symptoms, or relapse signature, and prompt management of them, if and when they occur. This of course depends on the establishment and maintenance of clear lines of communication between Wendy, her family and the involved carers. Her symptoms are most likely to occur during times that Wendy experiences as stressful. Tensions within families often cause positive communication to break down or sometimes cease. This can often lead to a difficult scenario for the sufferer – social isolation and loneliness. These are the conditions that, together with stress, are most likely to exacerbate the illness. A paradox can be that the sufferer is often unable to recognise, or unwilling to admit, that anything is wrong until they are immersed once more in the illness.

5.7 PERSONALITY DISORDER – DENISE

Preamble

The DSM-IV categorises and describes several types of personality disorder. The types are briefly as follows (American Psychiatric Association 1994, p. 629):
Cluster A: Paranoid, Schizoid, Schizotypal
Cluster B: Antisocial, Borderline, Histrionic, Narcissistic
Cluster C: Avoidant, Dependent, Obsessive Compulsive.
Gelder *et al.* (1999, p. 78) distils this into a list of general characteristics:

- Anxious, moody, and prone to worry
- Lacking self-esteem
- Sensitive and suspicious
- Dramatic and impulsive
- Aggressive and antisocial.

You will find, as a student, a wide range of opinion among experienced mental health professionals as to how this group of people should be cared for and treated, if they should be treated at all. Some will tell you that they cannot be treated, only managed. Your first experience of caring for a person with this diagnosis will probably be memorable and may cause you to understand this ambivalence, depending on how you are affected by the experience.

Profile

Denise is 22 years old. She has had many short-term jobs since she left school. She seems unable to settle in employment for very long. She had a brief stay in a psychiatric hospital when she was 18 and discharged herself against medical advice. The reason for admission at that point was a series of minor self-harm incidents followed by a relatively serious self-poisoning attempt. She rang her boyfriend at the time and he called an ambulance. She has been admitted to a local psychiatric acute ward because of another self-poisoning incident. The admitting nurse notices scratches on her wrist and both forearms. During the physical examination by the doctor the nurse also notices scabs and scratches on Denise's abdomen, as well as several tattoos, although these are not unusual on many females of her age.

During the admission interview Denise is surly and un-co-operative. Her eye contact is sometimes averted and sometimes threateningly direct. At least, this is how Jane, the admitting nurse, experiences it. Over the next few days Denise makes her presence felt on the ward. She is constantly demanding to go, although she doesn't say where. Apparently her relationship with her parents is very stormy. She says she hates her mother and her father is 'a bastard'. She has two other siblings who have nothing to do with her, she says.

Because the incidence of Denise's demands is increasing drastically and because she says that: 'Next time I'll do it properly', her consultant decides that a Section 2 is in order so that she can be detained on the ward for assessment, and treatment if necessary. This immediately causes Denise to become even more threatening and disruptive. The staff are involved in two separate restraint incidents over a weekend. As well as this, Denise has verbally threatened other patients, thrown crockery around and kicked the ward doors on several occasions. Many of the staff are becoming tired of her demands and behaviour, as are some of the other patients. This is a well established phenomenon. Visitors note that there is an 'atmosphere' on the ward.

Pathway through personality disorder

Jane tries to sit with Denise to get some understanding of why she is behaving in this way.

> **Jane.** Denise, could we have a few minutes together? Is that OK?
> **Denise.** Can I smoke in there? (*She points to the room that Jane is opening up for them*)
> **Jane.** No. Let's go in the day room. That's quiet at the moment. (*She notes that Denise is chain smoking and has a very slight tremor.*)

Even this brief interaction is full of potential difficulties. Jane is highly aware that Denise is very volatile at the moment. It seems risky to refuse her request to smoke in the small room. To acquiesce at this point could, however, mean continuing difficulties with rules and other boundaries. The ward team is highly aware that any 'breaking of ranks' seems to cause more difficulties, rather than less, with Denise. For example, during the night the nurse in charge escorted Denise off the ward for some fresh air. Denise now makes regular and noisy demands to do the same again, regardless of other pressures on the nursing staff.

It appears to the new student, Sharon Green, that Denise doesn't seem to have any understanding of what the nurses have to do. She seems very selfish and self-centred. A 'good turn' seems therefore to have turned into another stick with which to beat the staff. By choosing another venue where Denise can smoke, Jane is trying to listen to, and respond constructively to, Denise's needs without disregarding them in the interests of what seems to be application of an authoritative regime.

> **Jane.** So, tell me how things are for you at the moment.
> **Denise.** I'm sick of this fucking place.
> **Jane.** What 's the worst thing at the moment for you?
> **Denise.** Everything. It's like prison. Why can't I go?
> **Jane.** The main reason at the moment is the Section. If you weren't on a Section you could go, legally, but to be honest I wouldn't be very happy about you going.
> **Denise.** You're just like the rest of them. You just want to keep me locked up in here. I've done nothing. You're all bastards!

140

Jane. The last thing I want to do is keep you locked up. I'll be delighted when you're going home for good. (*She says this with no irony*.)
Denise. So you can't wait to see the back of me?
Jane. No, I'll be happy when you seem well enough to go.

Jane notices this characteristic of Denise, she seems to twist the words you say around to mean something quite different, usually negative.

Denise. There's nothing wrong with me.
Jane. So, talk me through the marks on your wrist and stomach. What's it all for?
Denise. I just want to go.
Jane. Tell me what's happening. I'm trying to help.
Denise. I won't do any more of this (*she points to the marks on her stomach*). I'm embarrassed. I look horrible.
Jane. That's a start isn't it? What makes you do it?
Denise. It makes me feel better. The pressure builds up like I'm going to explode, so I cut. I see the blood. I can feel the anger coming out of me, then I calm down. I feel better.
Jane. What do you think about coming to tell one of us next time you feel like you're going to explode. We'll try to talk you through it. That's if you really mean that you want to stop.

Here Jane is trying a gentle challenge try to test out Denise's commitment to change.

Denise. I don't know if I can. I can talk to you. You seem to understand me more than those others. At least you listen to me.
Jane. Good. Let's give it a try?

Jane feels that she has made a breakthrough. At last the hours of time and patience that she has invested into the relationship have started to pay off. Denise has started to relate in a more considered, adult, way. She seems to be more reasonable. This has all been achieved in an atmosphere of resistance and frustration on behalf of some of her colleagues. A small number of them have openly stated in hand-over that they think she is 'a waste of space ... not really ill ... taking up a bed'. Others have as little to do with her as possible. Jane wonders if Denise actually picks this up.

At handover next day, Jane hears that Denise has again been 'disruptive and demanding' overnight. She smashed crockery in the ward kitchen when one of the health care workers asked her to go to bed. Also small scratches have been seen on her wrist. Apparently she has cut herself with the ring pull from a drinks can.

Jane feels frustrated and resigns herself to another difficult shift. What's happened to her 'breakthrough' she wonders?

Jane. Hi, Denise. Tell me what happened last night to you?
Denise. That bitch Sharon asked me to go to bed so *I* showed her. She doesn't push *me* around.
Jane. What about the cuts on your wrist?
Denise. I did that afterwards. It helps me feel better. Like I told you.

Jane. You didn't ask anyone for help?
Denise. They're all useless on nights. You're the only one that listens to me.

Jane carries on the dialogue a little longer. She is trying to remain 'adult' and not get upset or frustrated by the seemingly endless repetitive sequence of self-harm and abusive incidents. She is constantly trying to reinforce the ideas that they have discussed about talking to staff when she feels frustrated. Jane is trying to model the Rogerian characteristics of genuineness (congruence), being accepting and being empathic. Sometimes, though, it feels really difficult and she starts to feel like a fraud. Inside she sometimes feels very unaccepting, unempathic, and incongruent.

She is pleased, however, that Denise still seems to feel that she is special: 'You're the only one that listens to me'. She has a sense of going around in circles, with no noticeable progress. Similarly, the conversation that they are having now seems to be going around in circles.

Later on in the day, Denise becomes abusive again to one of the other patients and accuses her of stealing her cigarettes. Jane intervenes and manages to separate them, although she has to call for assistance. During this incident Denise is abusive towards Jane. She addresses Jane as if there is no relationship between them at all. It is as if Jane is just one of the other staff. It feels to her as if all her efforts to help Denise have evaporated. Later, Denise is found to be missing from the ward. There is no news of her by the time Jane goes home.

Next day she arrives at work to discover that Denise has returned to the ward voluntarily. She had been drinking, had taken a small number of painkillers and cut herself across her upper thighs. Some of Jane's colleagues are making comments like 'Shame she didn't make a better job of it'.

Jane is starting to feel very isolated. She feels that she has to accept that some of her colleagues will never agree that, underneath the sometimes unpleasant surface, Denise is a very tortured and unhappy person. The nurses who feel they can work with Denise had decided that the only way that they could help Denise was really to work as a team. But already the team is split.

It looks as if Denise has been quite powerful. She has tried to make a small number of the nursing team feel that they are special and that they have a different relationship with her from the other staff. Jane thinks that this was actually true in her case, and that she *had* got a special relationship with Denise, but she is not sure what happened to it.

Jane. Hi, Denise. Can we have few minutes?
Denise. What for?
Jane. I just feel that we seemed to be getting somewhere with you recently but then it all seems to slip away and we go back to square one.
Denise. Everybody hates me on this ward! You're all the same – two faced. Nobody cares about me!
Jane. Well think about the number of times that I, and some of the others, have spent time with you trying to help you change things for yourself.
Denise. Fuck you, what do you know about anything?

Later that day, Denise tells Student Nurse Sharon Green that she has swallowed some glass she had powdered down from perfume ampoules. Denise now tells

Sharon that she is the only one she can talk to. Sharon is really pleased. She ponders: 'Just think, all the experienced staff on this ward and Denise thinks that *I'm* the only one she can talk to.'

Meanwhile, Jane decides that the only way that she can manage this kind of relationship with patients like Denise is to not become so involved, not to think that she is 'special' and to keep more of a distance. She then realises that she is becoming like some of her other colleagues who think that the best strategy is not to engage with patients like Denise at all, unless they really have to. Jane feels lost.

Denise now asks Sharon if she can talk to her 'in private.'

> **Sharon.** Denise, you wanted a word?
>
> **Denise.** Yes – could we go in here so no one listens to my business? (*She points to a small room away from the main day area.*)
>
> **Denise.** I want you to ring my social worker and ask her to speak to my consultant. I want to swap to another consultant anyway. I'm fed up about the treatment I'm getting in here. Well – lack of treatment. Nobody is helping me. Everybody ignores me. I might as well be back in my flat. Anyway you're the only one that listens to me in here. When can you do it? You won't tell anybody, will you?

Sharon feels instinctively that this isn't right. She knows that Denise is a 'sectioned' patient. Every patient has a right to request a different consultant. She is aware that lots of her colleagues do seem to ignore Denise, or at least have very little to do with her. Some of her colleagues think that Denise shouldn't be on the ward anyway, that she is a lost cause.

Part of Sharon feels sorry for Denise. She has had a difficult life, if everything in her notes is true. Now she's in hospital and having a difficult time as well. Sharon decides to contact the social worker and put the idea to her that Denise wants to change consultants. After this meeting Denise never mentions the request again. It's as if she has forgotten all about it. She also behaves in an off-hand way towards Sharon. Sharon finds this rather strange. What happened to 'You're the only one who listens to me?'

A few days later Sharon is sitting in on a care review meeting requested by Denise's consultant. Also attending are Denise, her social worker, a junior doctor, a psychologist, an occupational therapist, Jane and another staff nurse. After Jane has reviewed Denise's care over the past few weeks, the consultant brings up the subject of her request to change consultants. Jane and Sharon's nursing colleagues look bemused. They don't seem to know anything about it. Similarly the social worker expresses her concern that the ward staff don't seem to know this. Denise looks at Sharon – 'You know all about it, don't you, Shaz?' Denise has never called her that before. The consultant is starting to look very annoyed. He says, 'The nursing staff seem to have a communication problem here.' The social worker nods agreement. Sharon blushes deeply.

The consultant tries to find out from Denise why she wishes to change. Denise says she doesn't want to talk about it. After the meeting Jane and her colleague are very angry with Sharon. It becomes apparent that Denise has orchestrated things deliberately. She is unhappy with her consultant and, apparently, all the care team. She seems to have targeted Sharon as being the weakest link, the most naïve and inexperienced member of the team. Denise has split her away from the team and made her feel 'special'. After the initial annoyance with Sharon, Jane and her colleagues realise that they need to be supportive of each other. The nurses decide to try presenting a more united front:

> Denise. Hi, Sharon. Could you let me have some painkillers? I've got a splitting head after that row I had with my social worker. She said I was 'swinging it' in here and not making any effort to sort myself out. Jane said I could have some.

Sharon goes to find Jane, who says that Denise has already had a couple of paracetamol. She also says that Denise had provoked the social worker into being confrontational. Sharon returns to tell Denise she is not able to have any painkillers. Denise storms off to ask the ward manager. He checks with Jane and again the answer is 'no'. The staff are at last being able to give Denise a united and consistent message.

Gradually, over several weeks, Denise's behaviour seems to mellow. She is less argumentative, calmer and more willing to accept that things will not always go her way. A month later her section finishes and she returns to being a voluntary patient. For a few days she remains quiet and amenable. Jane has taken advantage of this window of opportunity. She is spending time discussing Denise's childhood days with her. She tries to understand what drives Denise to be so difficult. Denise seems able to talk about this for short periods then she becomes distracted and upset. She seems resentful towards both her parents, but especially her father. She goes out shopping one weekend. Shortly after her return she is discovered in one of the toilets cutting her legs again. Sharon finds her. When she has cleaned Denise's wounds they talk:

> Sharon. Why the setback? You were doing really well.
> Denise. It's all this talk about my parents. It winds me up. It's that Jane, she won't leave it alone. I'm reporting her to the consultant and the hospital manager. She breached my human rights. What I told her was private and now she's going around telling everybody. The whole ward knows my business.

Sharon has already heard that Denise has been telling some of the other patients about her childhood, so it is Denise herself that is spreading this information. The next day when Jane comes in Denise is verbally abusive towards her and throws an ashtray at her. The consultant decides to discharge her. She is an informal patient and the work that the ward team are doing seems to be constantly sabotaged by Denise. Some of the team say they could see that coming. After all, 'personality disorders are untreatable'.

A few months later Denise is re-admitted to the same ward. She has been assessed at the local police station by one of the court diversion mental health nurses. Apparently she has been threatening to kill a neighbour and last night attacked him with a brick. The assessing nurse contacts the consultant and he reluctantly agrees to have another try with Denise. She is admitted informally again. Jane asks if she can be Denise's named nurse. She'd like to pick up on the work that she did last time, even though it was very difficult. None of the other staff seem very keen to take over the role, anyway.

Jane. Hi, Denise. Sorry to see you back again
Denise. I bet you bloody are
Jane. No, I really am. I hoped you'd do OK when you went last time.
Denise. Yes well it's all gone wrong again, as you can see.
Jane. I wondered if we could do some work on the way you manage situations outside. It looks like you've been struggling a bit?
Denise. Yeah, whatever you say.
Jane. So what happened on this occasion. How did an argument with a neighbour get so out of hand?

Denise tells her story. Jane struggles with this. How much is true, how much is a product of Denise's imagination? Is she being manipulated already? Jane tries to be accepting of Denise, even though their past relationship has been fraught. She tries to accept what Denise says as a truth – Denise's truth. She listens in a quiet, respectful way, even though Denise is very animated throughout. After about an hour, Denise is starting to slow down. Already Jane feels worn out. Listening is still surprisingly tiring. Denise is blaming her parents, the hospital staff, her consultant and social worker, the police, and most of her neighbourhood, for the situation she is in. Jane tries something that she has never tried before:

Jane. What do you think you've learned from all this?

Denise looks aghast.

Denise. *I* don't bloody know. *You're* the nurse – you tell me!
Jane. I mean, what does this seem to tell you?
Denise. That I can't go on like this – and nobody likes me.
Jane. What makes you say that no-one likes you?
Denise. Everybody's against me, even in here.
Jane. On a good day, I think you're OK. You got on with Sharon OK, didn't you, after that glitch with you saying you wanted to change consultants? Some people find you hard work, but they haven't gone to the trouble of trying to get to know you a bit. Towards the end of the time you were here last, you made quite a few friends here, didn't you?
Denise. A few people started to talk to me sometimes. Sharon was nice, she did try for me. You seem to put up with me too. But no-one else bothers.
Jane. So what do you think started people talking to you last time?
Denise. I was interested in a few of them. I wanted to know how they were. They seemed unhappy or sad. They didn't annoy me.

Jane is trying to help Denise look at the occasions when she doesn't feel quite so attacked and negative. She tries to help Denise see that she does have some influence in how other people are with her. She pursues this style of intervention over the next few weeks. The subject of how Denise will manage in the future is gradually introduced by Jane:

Jane. When you leave here, what do you have in mind to do?
Denise. I don't know. I'll be going back to where everyone's out to get me, I suppose.
Jane. Over the past few weeks we've looked at the possibility that everyone is

out to get you. You've decided that it can't really be true, haven't you? So how come it still applies to your own neighbourhood?
Denise. It can't, but there are people there who don't like me.
Jane. Who are they?
Denise. The bloke two doors away. He never speaks.
Jane. Who else?
Denise. No-one ever phones.
Jane. That's a bit different isn't it?

Jane continues to gently challenge Denise's perception of her situation, with limited success. Denise is resistant and maintains her version of her situation that she is surrounded by people who are trying to get her, and that anything bad that happens to her is always someone else's fault. Denise still occasionally has outbursts where she becomes verbally abusive, but they seem to be reduced in frequency and intensity at the moment.

Summary of skills used

Denise, with her label or diagnosis of 'personality disorder', is seen as being one of the most difficult and challenging group of patients or clients. This is often to do with their struggle to relate to other people, which manifests itself as manipulative, power-seeking and inconsistent in its presentation.

Even though Jane tries a different approach with Denise during the second admission she consistently, through both admissions, uses a range of rudimentary skills.

- Jane really listens to try to understand what Denise is experiencing. This is likely to be particularly difficult because of the resistant nature of many people like Denise. It will feel like a fight just to listen.
- She is approachable, although the consequences of this with Denise is that Jane may be targeted for attention. Jane would have to very clear about boundaries of their interactions and meetings.
- She invests much time in slowly and consistently creating a rapport. This is likely to take a much longer time than is often experienced. If it happens quickly, it is probably superficial in its depth.
- Jane uses an open style of questioning. This is likely to be met by lots of resistant 'Don't know' and other methods of avoiding engaging with helpers (see also section 2.12).
- She attempts to be accepting and tries to not show any judgement. She experiences judgements inside her head, but these are never revealed.
- Jane tries to be empathic. This may again be met with more resistance than usual. The empathic attempt may be very accurate but Denise is likely to deny this.
- She attempts to create a therapeutic relationship. In this instance Jane would need to constantly question what that actually was. Supervision may help her with this.
- She helps Denise to reflect on how she appears to others. She would attempt this by giving her feedback, but she would need to be very thoughtful about how she does this. Her aim is to enhance her sense of self-awareness. The probable small impact that this will make may help Denise to be more

146

accepting of criticism from others, as this is an area that she finds especially difficult.

- Jane will be sensitive to the throwaway things that Denise says (see also section 2.15). These may contain truths about Denise that she is trying to disguise
- Jane uses Socratic questioning to help Denise work out things for herself. This is useful with personalities like Denise as they have a predisposition to blame everyone but themselves. It is necessary, therefore, for Denise to be helped to work out her own answers to her life's difficulties

Summary of approaches used to make up strategy

It is *essential* that Jane uses a collaborative approach. She will be very aware of needing to take an adult approach consistently. She will try to be person-centred, in terms of being empathic, congruent and accepting.

Prognosis

There is still some suggestion that people with personalities like Denise are not suffering from a mental illness and are therefore not treatable: 'The diagnosis can often be used as a derogatory label for patients we do not like or who do not get better' (Bloye and Davies 1999, p. 63). Rather than become involved in that debate, which is well covered in other texts, we will assume that Denise is suffering from some kind of mental disorder.

You will meet people like Denise during your mental health nurse training. They will often be patients in institutionalised settings. Part of the remit of this book is to indicate the ways you might try to engage constructively with this kind of person. If you go along with the idea that people like Denise of this world are untreatable, then what do we do for her, and with her, while we are nursing her?

Discussion point

What does untreatable mean?

You may have the uncomfortable experience of seeing Denise many times in several different care settings. All the while she is likely to be demanding, to seek and succeed in getting lots of attention from both carers and fellow patients. This attention does not seem to bear any fruit. You may find yourself going around in circles and having the feeling that she is not moving in any direction positively. You will probably be experiencing similar feelings to many carers before you, including, perhaps, her parents, teachers, friends, colleagues, and so on. This latter idea gives a flavour of the prognosis. It is not positive in the short term. To improve Denise's outlook needs a huge investment of care from our health services, and then there is no guarantee of a positive outcome.

Discussion point

What does a positive outcome mean in this context?

This is not to suggest that we should not try to help Denise and people who are like her. What is clear is that there are reasons, both historical and financial, that this is likely to remain a 'sticking plaster' area of mental health care, although there are some examples of effective treatment of personality disorder (Gelder *et al.* 1999, Stuart and Laraia 2001, Carson 2000).

5.8 ORGANIC ILLNESS IN THE OLDER ADULT – JIM

Preamble

Dementia is often an illness of such slow, insidious onset and gradual progress that it may be unrecognised for many months or even longer. In this sense it has similarities with other mental illnesses, such as depression or early-onset schizophrenia, where it is hard to tell the start of the illness from the end of the person's usual normality. Families may 'accept deterioration as normal, or fail to notice because the sufferer restricts his life-style so that deficiencies are concealed' (Evans 1982, cited in Brooking *et al.* 1992). Sometimes, concealment may be deliberate or a consequence of initial denial.

The changes associated with ageing are subject to considerable individual variation due to a mixture of inherited, environmental and life-style factors. Ageing certainly increases vulnerability to injury and disease but it is often a mistake to assume that all the effects of disease and physical deterioration in old age are inevitable.

Mood disorders may become more enduring in the elderly and take longer to respond to therapy, but full recovery is still achievable. Capacity for new learning may be diminished and problem-solving ability less efficient (and the consequences of these tendencies are often increased by persistent low mood). But severe memory impairment and confusion are not inevitable accompaniments of old age, although the incidence of brain disease rises steeply with increasing age.

The medical term 'dementia' refers to a group of related disorders characterised by progressive and irreversible changes in brain tissue that result in short-term, and eventually longer-term, memory loss.

The term 'demented' is stigmatising, as it is often used in everyday speech to imply somebody seriously deranged and possibly dangerous. For the sufferers of this type of illness it actually means extreme forgetfulness, confusion and disorientation. Memory for language is affected, so that meaningful conversation becomes seriously restricted. This in turn causes further frustration, anger, loneliness, sadness and fear, since in the early stages of these illnesses (and perhaps beyond), sufferers are often all too aware of the loss of their faculties: 'If we acknowledge that people with dementia will be experiencing at least one and probably many more feelings associated with loss, we can approach everyday tasks differently' (Wareing and Assey 2001).

'Senile dementia' (perhaps even more stigmatising) describes the illness when it occurs in people over the age of 65 and 'pre-senile dementia' when it occurs in people under this age. There are a variety of disease and degenerative processes that precipitate the syndrome of dementia, of which one of the commonest is arterial decay (arteriosclerosis) in the brain, resulting in leakage and clotting of blood that leads to localised death of brain tissue. This is often known as multi-infarct dementia and takes the form of a series of 'mini-strokes'.

Another common form of dementia is Alzheimer's disease. This is a degenerative disorder, of unknown origin, leading to the death of brain cells, which appears to take the form of greatly accelerated normal ageing. The rate of deterioration caused by the illness can be extremely variable – between 5 and 10 years (Hart 1990, cited in Wright and Giddey 1993) – but typically the brain will shrink until it no longer has the capacity to effectively regulate the autonomic nervous system controlling breathing, heart rate and kidney function, so death results from failure of one or more of these systems. 'Alzheimer's' seems to be a more socially acceptable term than 'dementia' and is often used loosely, by the public and professional carers alike, as an umbrella term for dementia of any cause.

True dementia, for which there are many causes, always implies an irreversible illness leading eventually to death. However, there are a number of related syndromes, which may be treatable, such as some brain tumours, acute confusional states, and 'pseudo-dementia', which is sometimes a feature of depression in some elderly people.

Profile

When Jim Coupland retired from his job as a train driver at the age of 65, he and his wife Marge sold the family home and bought a bungalow 60 miles away in their favourite seaside resort. Their three children were all in their thirties and living away from home by the time of Jim's retirement. All the family approved of the move to the coast, as it gave the excuse for regular trips to the seaside for the grandchildren. Marge's sister had been living there for many years with her husband. Jim and Marge had regularly taken holidays in the town and had a small circle of friends already established.

Marge started to become aware of a change in Jim, a few months after his 76th birthday. She had noticed that he was doing less around the house and garden but thought that this was just natural slowing due to age. He seemed more forgetful about little things, especially things she had told him about that she or other members of the family were planning to do. He was waking more often than usual at night. On a couple of occasions he had got dressed at one or two o'clock in the morning and had seemed astonished when told how early it was, but had come back to bed.

Marge had suggested that he go to the doctor's and ask for a prescription for sleeping tablets, but he had dismissed the idea, saying a large whisky would do him more good.

There were several occasions when she became rather irritated with him, and Jim too was often bad tempered and 'sulky'. However, this was only an exaggeration of the usual ups and downs of their relationship over the years. Most of the time Marge enjoyed his companionship and would make a joke of his absent-mindedness. She noticed she was having to do more for him and was sometimes astonished by how long it took him to do very simple tasks, like putting on his shoes and coat, when they were getting ready to go out together. On one occasion she had to fetch his shoes and hand them to him, and then help him on with his coat, several minutes after he had promised to be ready. He had also developed a tendency to sit staring at the same page of the newspaper for over half an hour. When Marge referred to a television programme they had watched together the night before, he sometimes appeared to have no idea what she was talking about.

One thing that did upset Marge was how he would become muddled about the names of the grandchildren, confusing them with his own children and in-laws. On more than one occasion he appeared to have entirely forgotten the existence of his youngest granddaughter, who was 4 years old. When Marge got angry with him he tried to make a joke of it, pretending he had just been 'winding her up'.

Marge eventually persuaded Jim to visit his GP. He seemed to be getting more and more forgetful and disorientated, eventually going missing for a whole day because he got lost in the town. After a long consultation the GP decided to refer Jim to a local mental health day unit.

Pathway into dementia/organic disorder

It was another two weeks after the events described above before Jim received a letter inviting him to attend a local day hospital three days a week, commencing the following week. Marge was invited to attend with him on the first morning.

During the two week interval Jim's behaviour had become rather more erratic, especially his sleep pattern and his tendency to ask repetitive questions. A prescription for sleeping tablets from the GP reduced the amount of disturbance for Marge at night but once the letter from the day hospital arrived the agitated questioning grew even more frequent. Jim seemed to be losing his ability to remember which day of the week it was (disorientation in time) and seemed to be under the impression that he was supposed to start attending the day hospital 'today' or 'tomorrow'.

Marge was very relieved when the day finally dawned and a car arrived to collect them, driven by a volunteer driver. On arrival at the day unit, a nurse called Bill introduced himself to the couple.

Bill explained that he needed to take some personal details from them for the admission form and then he needed to ask some questions about Jim's recent health and tell them what went on at the day hospital. Jim interrupted before he finished the sentence, saying that his health was fine and that he kept fit walking several miles every week.

> **Bill.** That's good. I understand you've been having a few problems with your memory, though, Mr Coupland. Is that right?
> **Marge.** Yes, he has.
> **Jim.** How did you know about that? Have we met before?
> **Bill.** No, we haven't. The letter from your doctor said so. That's why he suggested you attended here for a little while at least, to see if there's anything we can help you with.

Marge was wondering how much Jim really understood of what was happening to him. She had been aware recently that his attention to detailed conversation was very erratic, and she thought he sometimes pretended to understand more than he actually did.

It is a recognised feature of dementia that in the relatively early stages patients are often adept at covering up the full extent of their difficulties. This is known as confabulation (Bloye and Davies 1999). Their superficial social skills are often well preserved and it is only when conversation is steered towards fine detail that gaps in memory become clearly apparent, for example, part way through the initial assessment:

Bill. OK, Jim, could you tell me the day and date today?
Jim. Er, well I would be able to, but I've not seen a paper this week, and I'm not bothered about the radio or TV. They're such a waste of time aren't they? How long is this test likely to take?

The initial interview at the day unit continues:

Bill. Jim – Is it all right if I call you Jim? Most people here are on first-name terms.

This demonstrates respect, a tentative approach, not making assumptions.

Jim nods and says 'Yes'.
Bill. I just need to check a few details. Can I ask you to spell your surname?

This seems like a basic question for information but as you would expect it can reveal much information about Jim. For example: Does he understand the question? Can he remember his name? Is he able to spell it? We would of course check if Jim had the ability to do this anyway.
Jim responds without hesitation and also gives his date of birth when asked.

Bill. And you live at 12 Maypole Gardens?

Bill notices that Jim glances at his wife before confirming this. He also looks to her to give their phone number when asked, saying he 'just can't think of it at the moment'.

Bill. Do you have any children, Jim?
Jim. Yes, two sons.
Bill. How old are they?
Jim. Oh, now you're asking ... you'd better ask their mother (*looking at Marge*).

This on its own would not indicate an organic illness. Bill is looking for clusters of signs before suspecting any diagnosis, rather than coming to any conclusion from what might be a lapse of the memory.
Bill is glad to observe that Marge hesitates before answering. Nevertheless it is part of our nursing skills to keep the informal carers involved in a respectful, non-patronising way. Relatives often easily fall into the habit of answering for people with memory problems, partly to save them from the embarrassment of continually having to say they can't remember and partly to avoid awkward silences. They have often got used to this kind of compensating in other social situations with the client. However, Marge is keen for Bill to realise the full extent of Jim's problem.

Marge. Oh, come on, Jim, you must remember how old your own kids are!
Jim. I'm a man, we're no good at remembering birthdays and anni ... anni ... anniversereries [*sic*]. (*He stumbles slightly over the word.*)

The verifying and recording of personal details is an essential ritual whenever anyone is admitted into any health-care facility, whether in-patient, day care or community services.

This initial encounter, which might be seen as a simple (though important) documentation exercise, can be used by an experienced skilled nurse as an opportunity to attain several different goals, and begin to meet several different sets of needs.

The nursing goals could be:

- To carry out as full an assessment of the patient as is possible at this stage, given that the relationship is new and therefore levels of trust are likely to be relatively low
- To develop a rapport
- To attempt to establish the start of a therapeutic relationship
- To support and reassure the patient realistically and honestly
- To establish constructive working links with the patient's relatives/carers
- To establish constructive links with other helping professionals.

The patient's and relatives' needs could be:

- Honest information – 'according to the recent Audit Commission report, even carers of people with dementia are often kept in the dark about the exact diagnosis' (Borrill 2000, p. 23)
- Realistic support
- Being told what is happening
- Being told at a level that they understand and can manage
- Being communicated with by carers who at least *try to* be empathic.

Some examples of how this might sound with another elderly client are as follows:

> **Relative.** The whole family's worried about Edna. What's going to happen? Will she always be like this?
>
> **Edna.** Don't worry it's just because I get so tired that I'm confused. I'm sorry you're all so worried. I'm becoming a burden, aren't I? Who's looking after Sooty (*Edna's cat*)? Has he been fed today?
>
> **Nurse** (*addressing both Edna and her relative*). Would it be possible for someone to check on Sooty? It's not clear yet what's going to happen. Not even the consultant could predict that. We need to take things one day at a time. There are more tests that we need to do with Edna and then we may be able to see how things will go. It won't do you any harm to get a little more rest. Does it look like you're a burden, Edna? Your family seem to really care about you.

Here the nurse has the difficult job of trying to reassure two people who are connected to the same situation but who have separate needs. The nurse's primary task is to reassure in this scenario. There is no point attempting to give any factual information other than what is likely to happen in terms of immediate plans for Edna. The only practical action apart from this is to ensure that Sooty is being cared for and then try to reassure Edna accordingly.

Returning to Jim and Marge Coupland: their immediate needs are to feel welcomed, respected, understood and accepted. They also need to be orientated to the purpose and routines, as well as the layout, of the day hospital.

In receiving Jim into care, the Health Trust is also accepting responsibility for Jim's well-being, under the common law duty of care, even before comprehensive assessment has really started. It is therefore imperative that an accurate record, of who he is and who his most 'significant others' are, is registered as soon as reasonably possible. Without such a record it will not be possible to co-ordinate and collate details of his previous health records and, in the event of any untoward incidents it would be essential to inform appropriate people without delay.

So verifying the accuracy of these details is one of Bill's priorities. It might be easiest just to ask his wife, but this immediately presumes that Jim is incapable of answering accurately himself and diminishes his status. Although this may sometimes be unavoidable in parts, it should be tentatively tested. 'Where possible, clients should be included in conversation rather than being left to keep up with it' (Forster 1997). It is Jim's admission (although Marge's needs are equally important) and every effort should be made to engage respectfully his fullest possible participation in any procedure, no matter how routine.

By trying to elicit necessary information from Jim first, Bill is also getting an initial impression of Jim's memory, mood, self-awareness and motivation. Future observations and interactions will be supplemented at times by more formal assessment, such as the so-called Mini-Mental State Examination, which will be discussed later.

Jim is also likely to be asked what he has been told about the day hospital. He may have quite a good understanding of why he has been requested to attend there, or he may not. He may remember bits of information from the GP and have some insight into his gaps in memory and erratic behaviour. It is important to give him the opportunity to state his own understanding of events leading to his referral before giving some explanation of how he will be spending his time at the day hospital and how they will be trying to help him. This initial interview will possibly be kept fairly short, so as not to overtax Jim's concentration, which could make him anxious and agitated. The unit doctor will need to have her own interview with Jim and make a routine physical examination. This may happen later in the day. Sometimes the initial meeting may be conducted jointly by a doctor and a nurse or other member of staff, or the admitting nurse may sit-in on the doctor's interview.

Both Jim and his wife should be asked if they have any questions, and these should be answered as fully and as honestly as possible. Decisive opinions about the medical diagnosis and prognosis should only be given by one of the doctors. This does not mean that a suitably experienced nurse cannot discuss the patient's or relative's fears, but the nurse needs to be careful to invoke neither bleak pessimism nor false optimism. For example:

Jim. Am I losing my mind?

It is not possible to give any honest reassurance to this question. The possibility cannot be denied, since dementia does rob people of access to their most precious memories and eventually even the knowledge of who they are. But it would also be too abrupt and ambiguous to say 'Yes, perhaps'.

Bill (*in a tone that indicates serious concern, and with direct eye contact*). Is that how it feels to you?

Answering such a question with a question like this may sound evasive and create an impression of unwillingness to answer directly. This impression may be minimised by the attentiveness of the non-verbal response. It is a deliberately cautious reply by the nurse, who may have been surprised by the question and is giving himself time to collect his thoughts. But it is also a potentially empathic response, in that it recognises and responds to the fear and uncertainty that prompted the question from Jim, and seeks to focus his attention on his feelings. Since a definitive answer is not possible at this point, the need for information cannot be fully met; but a show of concern for his emotional turmoil may help Jim to feel supported and a little less alone.

At this stage it would almost certainly be only a provisional diagnosis of possible dementia. Other possible reasons for Jim's recent problems need to be assessed and investigated first.

The couple may or may not have been told a provisional diagnosis but even if they haven't they may have their suspicions. An opportunity to discuss it with someone perceived to be both sympathetic and knowledgeable, and perhaps with more time than the doctor, may be seized upon by patients or relatives. However, the nurse must stress that it is too early to be certain of the diagnosis. It cannot be overemphasised that this is an extremely delicate area and definitely not one for the beginner nurse to be drawn into. Nevertheless it is important to understand the principles of skilled responding on such a topic.

A possible conversation could go as follows:

Jim. I seem to be ... not remem ... remember ... not remembering so much. ...I do stupid things. ...Senile – is that what you call it? I'd rather know if it is. The doctor wouldn't say. What do you think?
Bill. It must be very worrying for you. The staff here will need time to get to know you, to make a thorough assessment. There may be lots of reasons why your memory has been poor.

At this point, Marge interjects: 'Is there anything you can do to make it better?'

Bill. It depends on the cause. It isn't always possible to be sure. We may be able to suggest things that will help you to compensate, Jim. (*Pauses for a second or two.*) You must be finding the uncertainty very difficult.
Jim. You hope it won't happen to you ... sometimes I feel OK ... my normal self. But then you ... you start to ... what you might .... Do you see what I mean?
Bill. I think I do. Jim, I know you are going to have lots of questions while you're with us. We'll try and answer them as best we can, when we can. We will discuss things with you. The staff here need time to get to know you. Can I make a suggestion? Would this be a good time to show you round the building and introduce you to a few people? Perhaps you could join in one of the group activities for a little while? It might help you settle in.
Jim. Activities? I don't know about that. I don't know anybody. What would I have to do? What about my wife?
Bill. Don't worry, Marge can stay if she wants to. You'll soon get to know people here. You'll be fine.

Summary of skills used

- The main professional carer, Bill, is welcoming and approachable. He needs to avoid being in any way intimidating. He is friendly, warm, and ordinary in a very specific sense (see also section 1.9). The first impression he makes will be very important to the new client and his wife. The process of assessment will be expedited and is likely to be more accurate if Jim and his wife are as relaxed as possible in a tense situation.

- Bill will be realistically reassuring. Again, the difficulties of doing this should not be underestimated. This is a very skilled thing to do. He will be as supportive as he is able, given this difficult situation.
- He is respectful. Bill will be as non-intrusive as possible, given that the nature of mental health assessment is always going to be intrusive by its nature.
- He maintains an honest approach. If the truth is difficult to face (*Will I get better?*), the degree of his honesty is tempered by caution (*We need to carry out a thorough assessment first. Then we'll be in a better position to tell you what you want to know*).
- Bill demonstrates an empathic attitude to both Jim and his wife. He tells them what is happening and what is likely to happen. He is informative.
- He sometimes gives them direct and clear instructions. He is directive.
- He occasionally suggests things to Jim and his wife. He is prescriptive.
- Bill is very careful in the way he handles the whole situation. For example, he avoids jumping to any conclusion about Jim and his wife. He allows them as much space as possible to talk. His whole approach is tentative.

Prognosis

There is at the time of writing no known cure for organic mental illness and little prospect of this as yet. There are suggestions that some medications can slow down the progress of the disease. When used together with thoughtful human interaction such as validation therapy, reminiscence therapy and resolution therapy, the results can seem to be encouraging, although opinion is divided on the effectiveness of these approaches.

It is true to say, though, that at the most distressing end of the spectrum, where the sufferer has in a few years lost the abilities to recognise their loved ones or carry out the most basic actions of self-care, there are practically no physical changes in the way people are looked after. Relatively recently, the idea of person-centred care (Kitwood 1997, cited in Kuhn and Verity 2002) has been adopted widely. The best that seems to be achieved is to look after basic nutritional and comfort aspects, with some intellectual or sensory stimulation as appropriate, together with a thoughtful and optimistic approach to personal interactions (Sammut 2003, Kuhn and Verity 2002). At its best this is very skilful work: 'the line between simple and patronising language is a thin one' (Armstrong and Wright 2002, p. 28).

The prognosis, then, is poor, and often the best we can do is to try to make sure that sufferers are as comfortable as possible and that their surviving relatives' needs are also acknowledged. They have already suffered one major loss even before the death of their poorly relative (Moyle 2002, Cutillo-Schmitter 1996).

5.9 SELF-DESTRUCTIVE BEHAVIOUR (DRUGS AND ALCOHOL) – JASON

Preamble

This is an area of care that will probably increase in size in terms of the number of people identified as needing professional mental health support. In most texts the areas of drug misuse, deliberate self-harm and alcohol abuse are reviewed separately. In this book they are treated in a similar way in terms of the beginner communication skills needed to start to engage with all three groups (see also the introduction to section 4.6).

Profile

Jason is a 25-year-old only son of middle class parents who live in a large detached house on the edge of a rural area. His father is a successful self-employed businessman. His mother works for the same business and is a director of her husband's company. Jason was a 'star pupil' at school until he reached the second year of his studies in the sixth form. He looked as if he would be following the family pattern of success and ambition until he was introduced to cannabis at a sixth-form party. He started smoking regularly and openly at home despite his parents' protestations.

This marked the start of his academic decline, as his parents would describe it. He seemed to lose all ambition. His studies were neglected. He couldn't or wouldn't concentrate, anyway. He eventually left school early with no A levels. His parents insisted that he find work, as they were unwilling to subsidise him sitting at home smoking and watching TV all day. His father reported him to the police for a series of petty thefts from their home. Eventually, Jason was asked to leave the family home and get a flat in the nearby town. Jason reacted to this by announcing that he was going to live in London 'with friends for a bit'.

He then effectively disappeared for two years, apart from the occasional phone call to ask for money. A month ago he turned up at his parents' house looking dishevelled. He had lost a lot of weight and seemed to have aged overly for his time away. Within days, despite his assurances to his parents, things started to go missing from the house. He had an argument with his parents, during which the police were again called to the house. Jason had been behaving in a very strange way, even for him.

The police called a member of the court liaison team, who screened Jason at the police station. He was subsequently admitted to a local psychiatric acute ward for assessment. During this process he was very threatening to the nurses and the admitting doctor. A decision was made to section Jason under the Mental Health Act (1983).

Pathway through self-destructive behaviour

During the next few days of his enforced stay on the ward, Jason is seen by the care staff as behaving in a generally difficult and disruptive manner. He kicks the ward doors on several occasions, demanding to go out to 'see some people'. He is very abusive to his mother, who visits on a couple of occasions. She decides not visit any more 'until he has changed his attitude'. The nursing staff observe him carefully to watch for any after-effects of withdrawal from drugs or alcohol. Jason is surprisingly co-operative when the nurses ask to do tests such as urinalysis for drugs screening. One of the nurses, Tina, seems to be building up a reasonably warm rapport with him. He is usually polite and amenable when she is around. The ward team decide that it may be helpful for Jason if she becomes his named nurse.

> **Tina.** Morning, Jason. Could we have a few minutes? There's something I want to discuss with you.
> **Jason.** No problem. What's up?
> **Tina.** The staff team wondered what you thought about me being your named nurse. Just on the basis we seem to get on OK. Perhaps we could review your care plan later on this morning?
> **Jason.** Yeah, that's good. I'm going outside for a smoke. I'll be back in a bit.

Tina goes through Jason's care notes, right from the day of his admission. She notices several themes over the past couple of weeks.

- Doesn't like being told what to do.
- Has been drunk on several occasions. No-one seems to know how he gets the alcohol. His friends, who visit, are suspected of bringing drink in to him.
- Becomes verbally abusive to the staff but has never physically attacked anyone.
- Is always very rude to both his parents when they visit. They seem to be visiting less and less.
- Is very flirtatious with the younger female members of the team.
- May have been taking non-prescribed medication. Again, it isn't known where this comes from.

Tina meets Jason to review his care plan. She tries to use a collaborative approach, where Jason is involved in his own care planning

> **Tina.** I see that you've been drinking on the unit several times and that you've been abusive to the staff as well. Perhaps this indicates that what we're offering you here isn't suitable to help you stop drinking. Any ideas how we could do it better?
> **Jason.** You could stop pushing me around for a start. You're all worse than my bloody parents. I get wound up and I need a drink or a smoke.
> **Tina.** When do you think we push you around?
> **Jason.** It's like you watch me all the time. None of you trust me, do you?
> **Tina.** It's difficult, isn't it? Since you've been here we keep finding that you have broken the agreement we made when you first came in. The bargain is only being kept on our side. That puts us in a very difficult situation as regards trust, doesn't it? I notice also, in your notes, that some of the staff find you very intimidating when you make sexual remarks to them.
> **Jason.** Oh, you mean Sharon.
> **Tina.** And others, not just her. So you see, you are making things difficult for us and difficult for yourself. What do you think you could do about all this?

Tina's intentions in this interaction are:

- To keep the conversation as person centred as possible – she is trying to keep away from an authoritarian approach as much as possible and attempting to respond to Jason's resistance against authority
- Constantly to put the locus of control (Barker 2000) back to Jason
- To use a Socratic approach, whereby Jason is given the opportunity to work out his own solutions
- To use open, non-directive questions.

There are major difficulties here around issues of trust and authority. These are worsened considerably because Jason is detained under a section. He has therefore very limited authority. Tina tries to make the most of very little.

She leaves him to think about their conversation and suggests that they meet again the next day. In the meantime Student Nurse Sharon Green is having a difficult time with Jason. She is in the final few months of her course and is now on the management module. She sees Jason walking past the office as she is trying to complete some discharge paperwork.

Jason. Don't speak then, Shaz.
Sharon. Sorry – I was thinking about something else.
Jason. About your boyfriend tonight? Lucky, isn't he?
Sharon. It's this paperwork, it's never-ending.
Jason. Yeah right . . . . What's his name, anyway?
Sharon. Just drop it, Jason, I'm busy. If you want to talk, I'll come and find you when I've finished this.
Jason. Can't wait!

Sharon pretends that she isn't bothered, by carrying on with the paperwork. But she is. She doesn't quite know how to handle Jason. It would be different if she'd met him outside of the hospital setting. She could tell him what she thinks of him. But she can't – he's a patient. She wishes that she hadn't committed to seeing Jason later on. She knows that if she doesn't talk to him later he will take advantage and cause even more trouble. She talks to Tina:

Sharon. I'm getting really fed up with Jason. He seems to keep picking on me and being very personal.
Tina. I know. I've had a word with him. It's not just you, but that doesn't really help, does it? Go and talk to him as soon as you've finished the discharge stuff. See if he can be reasonable with you. I gave him a lot to think about yesterday in terms of his treatment package. You could ask him about that – if he's thought of any way forward for himself?

Sharon goes to find Jason half an hour later, but he is missing. By the time she goes off duty he still hasn't returned. Four days later he is returned to the ward by the police. Apparently he went to London to contact his 'friends'. One of them rang his parents who then told the police. He is in a bedraggled state and again smells of drink. A drugs screening shows traces of cannabis and amphetamines.

Sharon sees that he is back on the ward when she goes on duty. She decides to go and find him as soon as handover finishes. She's got to learn to deal with this, as she's nearly qualified. The interaction with Jason is still uncomfortable. He really knows how to intimidate her. Then there seems to be a turning point:

Jason (*sarcastically*). I bet you were *really* worried when I went missing.
Sharon. I was, actually. You don't seem to have much control over what you are doing. You seem to be lost. I was worried.

Jason looks slightly shaken.

After several weeks, Jason is discharged on condition that he is referred to a specialist substance abuse worker, Liz. He agrees to this.

The approach that Liz takes is different, for several reasons:

- The setting has changed.
- Jason is no longer on a section – the locus of control has changed
- Liz is more in a position to let Jason take responsibility for his own actions. This is sometimes difficult in the institutional setting.

Summary of skills used

The main professional carer is Tina. Throughout the story above she demonstrates the following skills:

- She is direct and honest. As with several of the other stories the difficulties of doing this should not be underestimated. It is very skilful to be able to do this. Sometimes it feels that being direct and honest can cause patients or clients to become upset. It is nearly always worse to avoid this. Becoming upset is sometimes part of the process of becoming well.
- She is confrontational, but gently. She tries to help Jason start to face the consequences of his actions, not just to himself but to others.
- She remains clear about where the process is heading and therefore what her intentions are. This comes from the plan of care, which would be a consensus of the care team plus Jason's input.
- Tina uses a Socratic approach together with an open questioning technique. This is so she can help Jason work through his problems in his own way.
- She reflects back interaction content using Jason's own language.
- Tina tries to be empathic with Jason. As above, it is important to keep trying.
- She is quite clear about boundaries in terms of what she expects from him and what he can expect from her and the team.
- Many of the clinical interventions are aimed at increasing Jason's self-awareness with a view to helping him see the impact he has on the lives of others. Tina gives him plenty of time to reflect and make sense of his situation.
- She is consistently accepting and non-judgemental.

Summary of approaches used to make up strategy

- Tina uses a person-centred approach
- She tries to be accepting and non-judgemental
- She is clear about her intentions
- She works in a collaborative way.

Prognosis

This is going to be greatly influenced by the connections that Jason makes outside the care setting. There is a great risk that he will constantly gravitate back to the social circle or culture that supports his self-destructive behaviours. The strategy that the professional mental health care team consistently uses, during every admission (there are likely to be several as long as he is considered to be treatable), is one of helping him reflect on the impact his behaviour has on others and trying to help him to help himself and find his own resolve. In this sense the prognosis is not positive.

5.10 'COMPLEX NEEDS' – PAUL

Preamble

A reality of mental health nursing is that patients and clients often have multiple causes and clusters of signs and symptoms that mix together to comprise an illness that is unique to them. Some of these people appear to be suffering from a combination of disorders that may be seen as separate in some texts and are more complex than 'dual diagnosis' (Stuart and Laraia 2001).

In this story the pathway through a combination of different, but blending disorders will be examined. A contemporary term for this diagnosis is 'complex needs' (Keene 2001, Beer *et al.* 2001). Beer *et al.* (2001, p. 171) describe this as 'a severe mental illness, mainly in the form of schizophrenia or bipolar disorder, and in addition, has one or more additional problems such as another mental illness, substance abuse, medical problems, homelessness, history of abuse or lack of social support'.

Profile

Paul is a 32-year-old divorced man. He has lived alone for three years. His second wife left him after a difficult, short marriage. He has a daughter by his first wife but he has no contact with either. He does not have a job at the moment but has had many different low-wage jobs in the past. He lives in a rented room in an economically depressed area of a large city. He has many contacts with similarly dispossessed people.

Paul has a long history of drink problems and drug abuse. He appears to suffer from what may be a tendency to bipolar disorder. He has periods of being over-excited, then this tails off into a mild-to-deep depression. He has had several admissions to the local accident and emergency department with drug overdoses. He has described episodes of hallucinations to his community psychiatric nurse. He sometimes feels that people are following him and are out to get him.

Paul seems to understand the mental health system well enough to have got himself admitted to the local acute unit several times over the last five years. He never stops long enough to be meaningfully engaged by any carer. Either he discharges himself against medical advice or he is discharged by doctors who feel he is not suffering from any clear and treatable mental illness. They have been known to reach the conclusion that he is being 'manipulative' and 'knows how to work the system'.

Pathway through complex needs

Paul is currently an informal (voluntary) patient again on the local mental health acute unit. Staff Nurse Sharon Green is his named nurse. She has been qualified a few months and, after a difficult start, she is growing in confidence. She meets with Paul a few hours after his admission.

> **Sharon.** Paul? Good morning. I'm Sharon, one of the staff nurses, and I'm going to be your named nurse while you're here. Could you spare a few minutes, as there are some things I'd like to talk through with you?
>
> **Paul.** OK. What do you want to say? Have you got any fags?
>
> **Sharon.** No but I'll walk down to the machine with you in a few minutes.

Could we talk? I'd like to have regular meetings with you to review how things are going for you while you're on this ward. We'll do it every other day. If there's anything you need in the meantime and I'm not here, see my colleagues John or Richard, and they'll help you. I see from the admission notes that you've been having a rough time of things. Our aim is to get you back home as quickly as possible, but only when you are ready. When that point comes our intention is to make sure someone keeps an eye on you until you are settled again. That will probably be someone from our community team. How does that sound to you?

Paul. OK. Have you got any fags?

Sharon is aware of some of Paul's chaotic past history. She is aware of the many diagnoses and labels that he is carrying. She thinks that she is being realistic about what she and the team can achieve while he is in hospital. She feels that the *after-care* package needs to be as carefully considered as the care that Paul receives *in* hospital. She is determined that Paul will be an active participant in his care rather than a passive recipient. She realises how hard this is going to be, judging by his lack of engagement during this first meeting.

Sharon's intentions as Paul's named nurse are:

- To state her expectations clearly
- To get a sense of Paul's expectations
- To assess his level of commitment
- To make it clear that he will be participating in his own care
- To signal that there will be support after he is discharged
- To assess whether he understands all or part of what she has told him
- To find out how difficult it will be to start a rapport with someone who seems to be able to 'work the system' and may be quite institutionalised in his views and expectations.

Over the next few days, Sharon notices that Paul spends long periods of time off the ward. Some of her colleagues are starting to say that he might as well not be here. He is on no medication. Paul's consultant wanted to see what he was like after a drug-free period (sometimes known as a drugs holiday). When he is on the ward he seems to keep a low profile. He is friendly, speaks when spoken to, and seems to enjoy the company of a small number of the younger male patients, who have a tendency to be more boisterous and occasionally troublesome to the staff and some of the other patients.

Some of these patients are suspected of bringing in drink or have returned to the ward under the influence of drink or drugs. A couple of them have been discharged in the past week as they were clearly demonstrating no commitment to agreed treatment contracts and boundaries. Sharon feels that the drug-free period will be helpful to Paul but that the influence of this group could be difficult. Paul does seem to be 'easily led' and easily distracted from agreed goals.

An example of this is an agreement that Sharon makes with Paul to be back on the ward for 8.30 each evening. She tries to negotiate this for several reasons:

- To assess his levels of compliance
- To ensure that he is not pulled into difficult situations with disruptive patients

- To make sure that he is safe and accounted for, given his past history of disappearing for long periods
- To see how capable he is of sticking to agreed contracts – this will be important to do now with a view to the future, when he is under the care of the community team

Two days after Sharon agrees this with Paul he is not back by the agreed time. He returns the next day just in time for his evening meal. When Sharon talks to him he seems preoccupied:

> **Sharon.** Paul, where have you been? What happened to our agreement about 8.30 returns? I've been worried about you.
> **Paul.** Yeah sorry.

He attempts no excuse and gives no reason. Sharon sees that he is flat in his affect and seems a little distant. She decides to concentrate on this and try to asses his state of mind

> **Sharon.** You seem a bit cut off?
> **Paul** doesn't answer.
> **Sharon.** What's been happening to you?
> **Paul.** I took some stuff. I met my mates – they gave me some stuff. Those feelings have come back again. I feel like I'm sinking into a tar pool. (*This is an image he frequently returns to when he is becoming ill. It is part of his relapse signature and is mentioned in his notes.*)
> **Sharon.** A tar pool?
> **Paul.** Black, sticky. I can't get out of it. There's that voice again, telling me I'm crap.
> **Sharon.** Whose voice is it?
> **Paul.** It's mine, but it's nasty.
> **Sharon.** That sounds terrible.
> **Paul.** I manage. I've had it so many times. I'm just fed up of it all. I'm never going to get rid of am I?

Sharon's initial mild irritation with Paul for so quickly reneging on his agreement is replaced by concern when she sees how low in mood and defeated he seems to be.

> **Sharon.** Well it's perhaps a bit early to be saying you'll never get rid of it. Your consultant prescribed a drug-free period when you came in. We'll have to wait a while until this latest lot clears out of your system. What was it you took and how much?

Paul is still very vague, and he seems really tired and low. Sharon decides to leave him to rest. She tells the other staff to keep an eye on him. He does seem to be very low in mood, so precautionary observations would keep him safe and perhaps help to reassure him a little.

The next day Sharon goes to see how he is. The night staff report that he has had a quiet night and appears to have slept all through the night, apart from a period where he got up, had a cigarette and then went back to bed. They say that, while he was up, he would not speak.

Sharon finds Paul lying on his bed staring at the ceiling. She notices that already the area around his bed is becoming more and more untidy. Old magazines that he's taken from the day room, a couple of CDs out of their cases and several pairs of assorted socks are all on the floor. A smell of poor personal hygiene hangs in the air. He is unshaven. His eyes look blank, almost as if he doesn't recognise her.

> **Sharon.** Hi, Paul. How's it going today? I hear you had a reasonable night, apart from getting up once. Did you sleep?

She tries to find out how he is, but it's hard work. Paul is not being deliberately vague, she feels. It seems a great effort for him to talk, as if he can't be bothered. Sharon feels that a more directive approach could be useful. She is aware at the same time of the pitfalls of being too directive and over-helpful. Paul is very vulnerable to being even more institutionalised. Already there is evidence that he takes on this role very easily. Hence his tendency to be re-admitted on a regular basis. The way he is while on the ward, amenable, easy going, quiet, co-operative, all indicate this tendency. If Sharon starts doing things for him, then is she reinforcing this? Shouldn't she be leaving him to do things for himself by prompting him?

Sharon is aware that some of her colleagues would take a harder line here and tend to leave him to his own devices for exactly the same reasons. Maybe they are right, she thinks.

She starts to prompt Paul to sort out his personal hygiene and his bed area.

> **Sharon.** Paul, I'll run a bath for you in a few minutes. You can shave at the same time. Let's sort out these socks and magazines. We'll have a cup of tea and a chat afterwards. Come on.

Paul is co-operative but very sluggish in his movements. He seems to be almost physically retarded. His verbal responses are vague. It is as if he has become disconnected from life on the ward. Sharon realises she is telling him too many things at once. She slows down and takes each step one at a time. She also goes to get another nurse to help her and keep an eye on Paul while he is in the bath.

During the discussions over the next few days about Paul's care, the nursing staff express concerns to Paul's consultant about the way his mood and general demeanour have slumped. A consensus is that Paul might benefit from a course of antidepressants.

Some staff feel that that an antipsychotic might be appropriate too, as Paul still occasionally mentions hearing his own voice in his head. He doesn't seem to find this particularly upsetting, though. It is almost as if he is resigned to it. The decision is made to defer on this. It is not clear whether Paul is experiencing auditory hallucinations or intrusive thoughts that feel, to him, like voices.

The staff are aware that the antidepressants may take between two to three weeks to start having any therapeutic effect, if they work at all. This means that Paul still needs close monitoring for several reasons:

- To ensure his safety
- To ensure that Paul is near to care staff at all times and doesn't leave the ward unless escorted
- To monitor whether the antidepressants are having any effect

- To be selectively and thoughtfully helpful while trying to maintain Paul's independence and reduce his dependence

Richard is Paul's associate named nurse. He decides to spend some time with Paul to try to carry on the process of re-assessing Paul's mental state, as agreed in his care plan.

> **Richard.** Hello, Paul. How are you today? You're looking a bit brighter – or is that my imagination?

Paul smiles weakly and engages Richard with eye contact, which at the moment is quite unusual. Richard notices that Paul's bed area is cleaner and less untidy, but it's not clear if this is a result of action by Paul, or Sharon still looking after him.

> **Paul.** Not so bad, thanks. These pills are making me feel a bit weird.
> **Richard.** Weird how?
> **Paul.** A bit light headed, but OK really.

Richard tries to reassure him

> **Richard.** Stick with it for a bit longer if you can, then we'll get them reviewed by your consultant. It may be that those feelings are temporary. If not, it might mean putting up with for a while, or adjusting the dose, or even the drug. But try to persist a bit longer.

Richard knows from past experience that there is no point trying to change medication until the person's system has had time to adjust, unless the person is in severe distress. Paul finds Richard's honest informed knowledge very reassuring and he feels confident to follow Richard's advice at the moment.

Richard then tries to assess how Paul is:

> **Richard.** Apart from that, how are you feeling?
> **Paul.** OK.
> **Richard.** What about that voice you tell us you hear?
> **Paul.** It's OK.
> **Richard.** Over the last week, how many times have you heard it?
> **Paul.** Once, last night, just as I was going to sleep.
> **Richard.** What did it say to you?
> **Paul.** It called me a bastard. It said I was crap – it always does.
> **Richard.** What did you feel? You must have been frightened.
> **Paul.** No, It always says that kind of thing. I'm used to it.

Richard discusses this conversation with Sharon after first checking with Paul that this will be OK. Even though this exchanging of information is understood and implied, Richard feels that it might help to encourage the continuance of what seems to be an open and honest relationship that is developing between Paul and the ward care team.

Sharon goes to see Paul to monitor progress.

> **Sharon.** Hi, Paul. What's happening with you?
> **Paul.** I'm fine.

Sharon notices that this is said with some ambivalence. It's as if he isn't fine at all.

> **Sharon.** You don't really sound as if you mean that. Convince me.

Again Paul looks at her with strong eye contact. The nurses are beginning to realise that, when Paul does this, contact is being established. It is a clear sign with Paul that he is engaging.

> **Paul.** These tablets aren't doing anything. The voice is still pissing me off. I feel lousy. I'm bored in here. I'm just looking at the ceiling. I don't want to see anyone, no-one comes to see me anyway. I'm just a bloody loser.

Sharon is surprised by this outburst of negativity

> **Sharon.** Could we look at those things one at a time? You seem to be more agitated than you were when you started on the tablets. I'll ask Dr Mason to call in to see you later today to try to sort that out. As soon as you start to feel better, one of us will start to go off the ward with you. It is true you are getting very cut off. That's partially because of you not moving much away from your bed area, and it's partially to do with people not liking to come to these wards anyway. They're not nice places to visit, are they? How is the voice still pissing you off?
>
> **Paul.** It won't go away. Every so often it chips in and starts to get at me again.
>
> **Sharon.** Does the voice remind you of anything? Is it saying words that remind you of anything?
>
> **Paul.** Yeah – sounds like my dad. Lucie (*his second wife*) said all that stuff as well. She used to call me a loser.

Summary of skills used

Sharon, the main professional carer in the above story uses the following skills:

- She is very honest and direct right from the start. As discussed above, this can bring its own difficulties but on balance seems to be the most effective way to be.
- Sharon is informative. She tells Paul what is happening and what will be happening in terms of his treatment plan.
- She remains professionally accepting and non-judgemental.
- Sharon tries to be empathic.
- She is very clear about boundaries. This will be difficult for Paul as it is something that he has not been used to.
- Sharon is clear about her intentions.
- She is gently confronting and sometimes challenges Paul about his attitudes and beliefs.
- Occasionally she suggests things to Paul – she is prescriptive.
- She is constantly trying to find out more things about him but not in an intrusive way. She is catalytic.
- It is important that she keeps in tune with how Paul feels about situations. She is cathartic
- She uses open questions to give Paul the space to think about things.
- Sometimes Sharon feels it is appropriate to be directive but usually her goal is to be empowering.

Summary of approaches used to make up strategy

Sharon uses a problem solving approach together with a person-centred attitude of acceptance, congruence and empathy. She is clear about her intentions and works in a collaborative way especially with Paul himself

Prognosis

This is very difficult to predict, especially given the layered nature of Paul's problems. As with Jason in the previous story, there will always be a pull back to his 'normal' social situation and environment, which may support and even encourage the very behaviours that cause him to regularly become involved in mental health services. He is not an unwilling recipient of this, if we note his tendency to quickly become institutionalised.

The strategy of the team will be to consistently present Paul with appropriate behaviours and boundaries, with perhaps, as appropriate, a problem-solving approach that will support him to find his own resolution of his difficulties. This would all be delivered supported by a person-centred philosophy.

6 PUTTING IT ALL TOGETHER. THE COMPLETE, EFFECTIVE, PROFESSIONAL MENTAL HEALTH NURSE

This section completes the circle so that the focus now becomes the reader rather than the patient/client/service user. Some of the material in this section concerns managing rather than coping in a job where the demands and expectations seem to be increasing exponentially (Malone 2003). This chapter is not about how to survive but about how to avoid getting into the situation where it feels as if your survival is at risk. The skills, techniques and ideas discussed in Chapters 1–3 are used for different purposes here.

6.1 LEAVING WORK BEHIND

This is a skill that usually develops as you become more experienced. At first, and perhaps often when you first qualify and the responsibility seems very heavy, it is difficult to disengage from what you have been doing for the last eight hours, almost regardless of the setting. You may experience doubts about having completed tasks, or worry about passing information on to people back in the clinical area or your base.

There are two courses of action here. Do something about it, or don't. Action will put your mind at rest, especially when you are reassured by one of your colleagues, who tells you that you shouldn't have worried and 'It's been dealt with'. A few more calls like this and you are more likely to get the feel of when it matters and when it doesn't, or at least when it can wait until tomorrow or the next time you are at work.

If you find that you are having difficulty disengaging from events at work and the problem appears to be worsening, then your supervisor or a respected colleague may be able to help. This is a matter of your perception of the relative importance of events to you. For example, you may be worried about a patient who has been discharged against medical advice. You have had a lot to do with their care. You feel a sense of personal investment. Once they have left your care there is nothing else you can do as a professional apart from give them the option of making contact with your care team if things go wrong again for them. The responsibility is in all respects with the discharged person as long as all reasonable attempts have been made by the different professionals in the team to constructively persuade the person to accept the care offered. If they still decide to discharge themselves then they are exercising the same rights that you have and that you value.

Certainly the inability to manage this kind of situation is dangerous to health and can lead to professional burnout. McLeod (1998, p. 301) suggests that 'the helper becomes caught between his or her own high standards and the impossibility of fulfilling these standards, and after a while is unable to maintain the effort and energy required in functioning at such a high level. This is the state of burnout'. Note that nowhere in this explanation is any connection made with length of service. It is to do with a level of personal commitment to try to achieve impossible goals. In this sense the ambitious new starter is very vulnerable.

6.2 RELATIONSHIPS AT WORK – UP, DOWN, ACROSS

Relationships with colleagues are consistently recognised by students (in my own experience as a mental health teacher) as being probably a more difficult area to navigate than relationships with patients and clients. Sometimes this has to do with the transience of the student–assessor relationship. Sometimes it is to do with institutionalised, negative or destructive attitudes that seem to be welded into the personalities who work in some clinical areas. This, by the way, includes the range of workers from domestic to consultant. Given the difficulties of tackling these problems on an individual basis, as a student or newly qualified nurse, and given that sometimes these well known situations are 'ignored' by nurse management, the worry that this can cause the student or newly qualified nurse cannot be underestimated. The solutions are almost always uncomfortable or unpleasant. This probably explains why they are so often avoided.

The preferable option is always to try to sort the problem out yourself. If we revisit the rudiments, some of the ones that can be most useful in these situations are:

- *Self-awareness – how do you appear to others?* Most students are keen and enthusiastic, eager to please and to make a good impression. Sometimes, though, they can be unmotivated, introverted, apparently lacking in initiative and unreliable. So perhaps you can use some of the above positive qualities to integrate yourself into the group of people you are working with for the next few weeks or months (or in some cases years). Never underestimate the power of making tea (and other work rituals) for your colleagues or taking on other more mundane tasks such as helping with the laundry. You will be surprised how much you can learn by looking at someone's unmade bed. Don't wait to be asked, offer to do it. During this process you are creating the opportunity to make the first contact with many other members of the clinical fraternity by offering them a drink. Next is the issue of your image or self-awareness. You have to find an appropriate level of keenness, tempered with human frailty such as tiredness at the end of a working day. Perhaps a degree of introversion can be easier for an established group of people to accept than a buzzing enthusiast who has apparently endless energy reserves.
- *Self-disclosure.* A little considered self-disclosure about other aspects of you that exist outside work can help you to integrate. You can demonstrate the ability to be a rounded personality rather than someone who lives and breathes mental health.
- *Timing.* As a student or newly qualified nurse you will want to, and need to, know a vast range of things. It is not only you, though. You will be regularly put in the situation of needing to know things on behalf of patients/clients and their relatives. This is because you may be seen as more accessible than some

other members of the care team who are more likely to be enmeshed in office-based work. Choose your time to deepen your knowledge. Prioritise what you need to know.

Discussion point

What might be the learning priorities for the newly qualified staff nurse? What do these priorities depend on?

For example, the situation when a relative asks you what the visiting hours are for the ward or when the consultant is likely to visit the ward is very different from not knowing the side effects of an SSRI. If you suspected a patient is suffering from medication side effects, your course of action is to ask one of the trained nurses (or a doctor, if available) to see them quickly, rather than trying to work it out for yourself, because in the meantime the patient may be in danger or discomfort.

- *Starting a rapport.* The skills needed here are no different from the skills discussed earlier in the book. Regard the target of your relationship skills as being the individual members of the care team. You are likely to have the same range of 'successes' as you have with the group of patients.
- *Ordinariness.* Be yourself. It is absolutely exhausting trying to be something that you are not. Being genuine will also help you keep in touch, and congruent with the person-centred philosophy of working, which is usable in many mental health settings in some form. Most people will respond to this positively and constructively.

6.3 YOU'RE THE BEST NURSE

These words may occasionally be said to you by a patient or client. Ask yourself what these words mean, coming from this particular patient/client, at this particular time, in this particular setting? Sometimes the patient/client saying this will mean it very sincerely: 'At this moment you are the person who is giving me what I want and what I need'. Often the reasons for this are that your colleagues are otherwise occupied, or they aren't prepared to tell this person what they would like to hear.

In some cases the person will choose you deliberately because they like the look of you, see you as a 'soft touch', or see you as someone who really will make time to talk to patients. Sometimes the person will say this to you to 'split' or separate you from your colleagues. The reasons for this are often devious. This separateness can be used against you in the future: 'Well, Jane (*you*) said I needn't keep taking these tablets because she doesn't think that they are helping me'.

The reasons people will say this to you, then, are many. In a mental health setting, consider the reward that person is trying to get by saying those words to you. Be careful. Sometimes it is prudent not to take such compliments at face value.

6.4 Relatives of patients and clients

A useful idea here is to remember that when you admit, or take on to your case load, any person, you are in some sense taking on their family as well (Gelder *et al.* 1999, Stuart and Laraia 2001). This doesn't just mean involved, supportive relatives and family members. If the father of a patient is dead, and was supportive when alive, it might be that he will be missed and add to the senses of loss and isolation of that person. On the other hand if he was unsupportive the effect might be that 'I survived and managed that, so I will survive this'. Whatever the perception of the patient, it is usually important to try to avoid nursing the person in isolation from the impact of their significant others. This applies whether these people are present or absent, alive or dead.

It will also be sometimes apparent that the relatives of patients/clients appear to be more mentally unhealthy than the person who is on your ward or your case load.

Relatives can be extremely helpful in supplying the pieces of the jigsaw that are missing, either knowingly or unwittingly. On the other hand they can appear to be interfering and can apparently cause exacerbation of the person's condition ('triangling'; Carson 2000). For example, every time Jake's mother visits him he is agitated for several hours after she has gone. The effective and creative mental health nurse would want to know the reasons for this. Some answers may come from Jake. Some answers may come from his mother. Other answers may come from more distant and less involved relatives. Other answers might come from your own observations and the observations of colleagues.

These answers, however, might be only part of the story. You may never access the truth, but it is important for the care of the patient that you make the effort. Whatever your views on the role of the relatives or family members in the care of people needing mental health care, you need them more than they need you, if you are to maximise the effectiveness of your nursing interventions.

6.5 Being professional

What 'being professional' means

'Being professional' means behaving in a way that is exemplary and representative of good nursing practice. It means being objective and honest. It means being considerate and doing things in your work setting that always put the patient first. It means doing all the above things on a basis of recent research-based knowledge (you will probably see this referred to as 'evidence-based practice'). These expectations are based on commonly accepted layperson's views of what we should do in the job of mental health nursing. Given the production-line pressures (Malone 2003) on nursing generally at the present time and given that this pressure is unlikely to lessen, where do these expectations leave us?

The NMC Code of Conduct sets out the professional practice guidelines for qualified nurses. Student nurses follow the same principles. According to the Code of Conduct, we are expected as qualified nurses to maintain confidentiality and protect the 'best interests' of the patients we care for. The Code of Conduct essentially covers the following professional areas:

- Respect for the client
- Obtaining consent
- Protecting confidentiality
- Co-operating with other carers
- Maintenance of professional knowledge and competence
- Being trustworthy
- Minimising risk to clients (NMC 2002).

A dilemma this might present

One important question that the above is likely to raise could be 'Where does confidentiality start and where does it stop?'

Jemma has just been admitted to the ward under a Section of the Mental Health Act. Her next door neighbour, with whom Jemma often has a cup of coffee, witnessed a scene where Jemma was apparently pushed into a police car and taken away. The neighbour rings the mental health unit and manages to track down the ward where Jemma has been admitted:

> **Neighbour.** I'm phoning up to find out if Jemma Britton is OK. I live next door to her. How is she? What's happening to her? (*The neighbour is enquiring out of genuine concern.*)
>
> **Nurse.** We are not able to tell you what's happening to her because of confidentiality, but I can assure you that she is being looked after and is safe. I will tell her you called if you like.

The nurse then tells Jemma that her neighbour has asked after her:

> **Jemma.** What the hell do you think you're playing at? How dare you tell her I'm here! You've no right to do that – what about my privacy? I'll have you all in court for this!

So here we have confusion and different perceptions of what is meant by confidentiality and the different values that different people put on it, depending on their roles in the story. The neighbour is rather bemused by the reticence of the nurse because at this point she knows more about the build-up to Jemma's relapse than either the professionals involved or Jemma's relatives.

The nurse does the best she can. She is trying to protect Jemma's privacy. If Jemma's mother had phoned, the nurse might have not have felt it necessary to be quite so careful (although she doesn't know that Jemma and her mother haven't spoken for six months). On the ward, once 24 hours has passed, Jemma's story has been heard by twelve nurses and six health-care assistants, two occupational therapists, a pharmacist and a couple of doctors. Her community psychiatric nurse and GP have also been informed about her admission. One of the above carers on getting home that day says to her husband:

> 'Guess who was admitted today. . . .'

All the above actions except the last are carried out in the 'best interests of the patient'. You will find that there are a wide range of opinions in mental health nursing as to what these are. Everyone has a view. Often, there is tension caused by differing views. This is not always necessarily the patient versus the carers. Sometimes the carers themselves will have opposing views as to what is in the patient's best interests. The nurses may find themselves involved in a battle of wills with an autocratic consultant as they try to advocate for what they see as the best interests of the patient. Again, a not unusual situation is for the patient to want something that the carer team sees as not in their best interests (Wright and Giddey 1993).

6.6 CARER OR POLICE?

You are likely to find yourself in this situation at some point in your career as a qualified nurse (Coombs 1996). There is a possibility that even as a student you may become involved on the periphery of it.

The incident usually occurs within an institutional setting. You have spent some time trying to develop a therapeutic relationship with a patient. Despite the best attempts of the care team, the patient starts to relapse. He constantly demands to go home. He leaves the ward and is brought back by angry relatives on a couple of occasions: 'Why can't you keep him here? You're supposed to be looking after him.' The consensus decision of the care team is to ask the medical staff to section the patient under the Mental Health Act so that he can be detained for assessment or treatment or both. The ward is understaffed and the nurses who have been working with the patient are constantly trying to negotiate with someone who does not want to listen to reason.

The patient is seen by two doctors and is eventually put on to a Section 2. The rights of the patient are read to him by his named nurse, who is part of the team that wanted to apply for the section. The patient knows this. He is angry with the nurse, as he feels let down and betrayed.

This creates one of the most difficult situations for both the patient and the nurses who are working with him. The patient does not know if the nurses are his carers or his custodians. In reality they are both. The only way to manage this is to consistently use the basic skills described earlier in this book. They will still be effective in terms of starting to re-establish something resembling trust, although this will undoubtedly be difficult.

Those basic skills are the Rogerian ones of:

- Attempting empathy with the person's situation
- Being accepting of the person's unhappiness/anger/frustration with the situation
- Being congruent or genuine in providing information on their situation.

What is described here is one of the most difficult tests put before mental health nurses as part of their everyday role. The tension is clear to see. How nurses handle this is down to their personality and the way they access the support that is available to them formally and informally. Certainly, a team of carers that has a strong sense of unity can manage these situations more effectively in terms of the impact on individual team members. Some nurses may be hardened to this or don't show it. Others may be more sensitive and upset.

For the beginner nurse a useful strategy would be, as always, to discuss the situation with an established member of the team whom you respect. Then go away and reflect on it. One day it is likely that a beginner nurse will be asking you the same questions.

At the time of writing, changes to mental health legislation are being debated that look as if the situations explored above could become even more difficult (Laurance 2003).

6.7 I'M REALLY FED UP

Sometimes it may be you saying this or thinking this. Sometimes it will be your colleagues saying this, or looking as if this is the way they feel. It is important that you listen to yourself and acknowledge these thoughts and the feelings that may be coming from them. Some questions you can ask to start to address this are as follows:

How long have I felt this way? Is it just today or is it longer term?

Sometimes the sense of being fed up can be around for months quietly simmering away. Sometimes it jumps up into your mind from nowhere. It is useful to try to figure out if your feeling is a reaction to some event today or recently, or if it is an accumulation of events and occurrences that have gradually worn away your enthusiasm and fizz. Also is this typical of the way you react to situations (life)? Are you reactive as a rule, or are you more thoughtful in how you respond to things?

What does 'fed up' mean at the moment?

Is it a dulling of your natural spontaneity? Does it mean you feel run down, burned out, slowed up? Can you catch your 'automatic thoughts' (McLeod 1998, Blackburn and Davidson 1990)? What do they tell you? How is it manifesting itself in the way you are both at work and outside work? Has anyone else noticed – your friends, colleagues or even your clients/patients? Are you functioning as usual or are there changes in the pattern of your life and habits?

Is a physical 'fed up' or a psychological 'fed up'?

Do you feel as if you are moving in treacle? Is it more and more difficult to get out of bed to go to work? Do you have difficulty going to sleep because you are constantly re-running the day's events? You are waking up in the early hours of the morning doing similarly? You wake up and as you realise it's time for work, your heart sinks? Is it a combination of any these?

Are there any identifiable triggers or causes?

If your response to this is 'I don't know', then this might indicate that some outside help could be useful to you. Try to find someone you can run these thoughts past.
  Some of the possibilities are:

- You don't like the job or the job setting any more
- Events there are causing discomfort for you
- You are not happy in your work role: it stretches you too much or not enough
- You are suffering from something physical – the aftermath of a cold, anaemia, poor diet, an injury or illness
- You are suffering from something psychological – anxiety, depression

- You are reacting to discomforting events outside your work, such as spiritual issues, relationship issues, financial issues, accommodation issues, and so on.

Mental health nurses are probably, in general, no more skilled at managing their own life events than any other members of the general population. Do not feel that because you work in mental health you 'should be able to manage'. Access to friends, family, colleagues, the right counsellor or your GP are just as important to you as to any other person.

How can I start to get through it or overcome it?

As you would indicate to any patient or client, this is difficult to do in isolation. As mentioned above, the most valuable weapon you can use to make maximum impact on your feelings of being 'fed up' is the help and support of another person or a small group of people. They don't even have to know that they are doing anything.

For example, you have been worrying about an incident on the ward. A couple of days ago, a patient screamed at one of your colleagues, Teresa. The action you took was to keep other patients away from the area while the situation was managed. This was your rational response. Your emotional response was to be protective towards Teresa. The patient was being abusive and making very cruel and personal remarks about her physical appearance. Nothing has been said since, as far as you are aware, to support Teresa. You are very uncomfortable about all this. You approach your colleague:

> **You**. I'd like to say, I feel really awful about what Eric said to you the other day. I left you to cope with him on your own. All I could think of was to get the others out of the way so you could deal with it.
> **Teresa**. What you did was spot on. I would have done exactly the same. It's not right that the other patients are exposed to that sort of language. Eric apologised to me the next day. You were off, so you wouldn't know that. He's done that several times before. It's just how he goes sometimes.

It looks as if your colleague has managed the situation herself, or at least there seems to be some sort of resolution to it. Whereas you are the one who has really been agonising about it. This example of 'off the cuff' impromptu supervision shows how usually your actions are at least OK and probably often more effective than you imagine.

6.8 IT'S NOT FOR ME

This can happen at anytime during your training or at any time during your career as a qualified nurse. A helpful strategy is to try to recognise whether this thought is a normal part of the way you think. Or is it part of a longer process of you being worn out by the job, or the course, or both, and its demands. Some people fall very easily into 'defeat' as part of their pathology: 'Nothing I do goes right'. This can be lived with/survived in a supportive atmosphere where your colleagues and friends and family will be able to point out to you that this slump is temporary and that in the bigger picture things aren't quite so bad as they feel at the moment. If you are a student it might be worth considering and getting advice on the possibility that you are studying for a branch of nursing that doesn't suit your needs and exploring the possibility of a change to another branch. Just going through this process sometimes helps to clarify what it is that feels 'wrong'. If you are a qualified nurse, then supervision (if available) could be the ideal place to clarify what you could do to start to sort this out for yourself.

6.9 Moving on to specialise

Some nurse students know what they would like to specialise in even before they start their training. Some are grabbed or inspired by a particular speciality during the course. Some are open-minded and remain so. Some are ambivalent and remain so. There are pros and cons to committing yourself to becoming a specialist. Some of the advantages are:

- Your focus on a relatively narrow field of expertise should mean that you have the potential to give more specialised patient care
- You will be able to find research that will help you maximise that patient care
- You will be able to carry out research to further the body of knowledge in your chosen speciality
- You are likely to be seen as having a higher professional status, even if this not recognised financially
- You may attract higher financial status.

Some of the disadvantages are:

- As a specialist you will not be meeting the broader spectrum of patients that a generalist would
- You may become bored or disillusioned with the group you are specialising in
- Your specialism may fall out of favour
- Deeper entrenchment into your speciality might mean greater difficulty in transferring to other fields.

Overall, there are probably more advantages than disadvantages to becoming a specialist. The personal characteristics you will need to demonstrate are commitment, enthusiasm, a creative approach and a passion for the speciality. The commitment will almost certainly require you spending large parts of your out-of-work hours building up your study CV. A degree is becoming common-place, study at master's level is not unusual and doctorate level commitment seems to be not far away. This gives you an idea of the commitment involved if you really desire to reach a high status in a specialist part of nursing.

It is possible to start planning and developing your career from a very early stage. Throughout your training you will meet people who will be willing and able to help you activate these plans. Be aware that, however quiet and introspective, or loud and extrovert, you are, you are being watched and weighed up by your trained colleagues. Many of them will be subconsciously asking themselves: 'Could I work with this student as a colleague?' Try to ensure that the answer they are coming up with is 'Yes'. You never know when or where you will meet people again in your future career – they tend to pop up in the most unexpected places.

6.10 Supervision

Supervision is often seen as a panacea for job satisfaction in nursing literature: 'The issue of clinical supervision is of great importance to all staff who are involved in the day to day care of patients. It is particularly important in areas of high stress where patients may be difficult to treat' (Beer *et al.* 2001, p. 311) It is 'a process of trusting enquiry' (Wright and Giddey 1993, p. 7). A positive relationship between supervisor and supervisee can considerably enhance the working experience of both, although the focus is of course on the supervisee.

The characteristics of this relationship at its best would something like this:

- There is high level of trust between the parties. It must feel that anything can be said in confidence, given the usual clearly understood exceptions to this such as apparent abuse of a power relationship.
- There is a high level of respect between both parties. It is a cliché, but this respect is earned and not bestowed upon either person. The respect can only be there if it is experienced as such by each person for the other.
- There is an agreed, and stuck to, regular arrangement to meet. It is contracted, in other words, not an *ad hoc* 'whenever it seems to be necessary' arrangement.
- Ideally, although the reality is often different in health care trusts, the supervisor should not be in a management relationship to the supervisee.

In practice, things can be different from the ideals reviewed above. Often there is a management relationship between the two parties and this is likely, even with the best will in the world, to affect the quality of the relationship and *possibly* impair its usefulness. In this setting the effectiveness of the relationship could be measured in terms of:

- Does the supervisee feel that their clinical practice can be constructively reviewed and critiqued in isolation from any management issues?
- Can their relationships with colleagues and patients/clients be similarly scrutinised?
- Can more personal, but still professional, issues such as countertransferences be aired?
- Can personal issues be discussed in view of their impact on the work of the supervisee? (see also Newell and Gournay 2000).

6.11 Debriefing

Beer *et al.* (2001, p. 313) suggests this as a way of managing after 'serious incidents'. All staff involved should be included. The session is facilitated by a senior person who was not directly involved in the incident. If possible, patients should also have the opportunity to attend a debrief.

This would be seen as entirely separate from individual supervision, but of course people may use supervision sessions to continue processing any unfinished business. The hope would be that any debrief would help people to manage the issues that come from serious incidents, given the sometimes traumatic nature of incidents in mental health settings.

6.12 I DON'T LIKE HER ATTITUDE

This is another difficult issue for you, both as a student and as a staff nurse. Occasionally, you will see practices and attitudes demonstrated by your clinical colleagues that give you cause for concern. This might be at several levels:

- You feel that the person has been 'unprofessional'. Before you do anything else, it may be helpful to re-read your copy of the NMC Code of Conduct. How is the attitude or behaviour of your colleague objectively unprofessional in terms of what you have read? Your next course of action could depend on this. Do you approach the person directly and challenge them about it? Do you talk to colleagues, either directly or obliquely? Do you discuss it with your manager? Do you talk it through at supervision?

- If the person is not objectively unprofessional but their clinical attitude disturbs you, what might this mean? This could be the time to turn around the accusing finger and point it directly at yourself with the question 'What does this say about me?' You might be surprised at the answer and you might not like the answer, but try to listen to it anyway. A positive supervision relationship can be tremendously helpful at these points in your career.

- The ideal course of action is to have a discussion with the person who is raising the concerns within you. This is easy to suggest but can be difficult to carry out. It can be an act of great courage to challenge someone in your work situation. You can try to predict the outcome of the challenge by rehearsing in your head what the likely results might be of your challenge. More often than not, your predicted outcome will not happen and you will be surprised – sometimes pleasantly sometimes unpleasantly.

- Ultimately your choices are probably one of three – do something, procrastinate or shut up. Which one you choose will be a matter of the balance between your courage and your conscience. This is a basic dilemma of many effective mental health nurses from time to time.

6.13 ROLL ON RETIREMENT

From the start of your career as a mental health nurse you will occasionally meet people who seem to be disillusioned, very cynical and who are 'winding down' to retirement. It can be disappointing to be exposed to this attitude, especially when you first start. At this stage in your career it is hard to understand how anyone can be disillusioned with caring for others.

Put in context. though, see for yourself how changeable, dynamic and difficult nursing is today. Consider that some of the more experienced nurses you work with will have seen the scrapping of, for example, the Mental Health Act (1959), asylum-type care, uniforms (but they are now coming back), widely used seclusion procedures, large-scale institutionalised care settings. They will have seen the introduction of the Mental Health Act (1983) (now being reviewed again) and community care, de-institutionalised practices, patient empowerment, and so on. Given the best will in the world to maintain the care ethos that was brought into the job when they were younger, it is no wonder that so many people yearn to stop doing the job.

And yet deep inside they are still often caring people. It is just that the outer shell has hardened. The way you can manage this is to have some empathy with, and understanding of, what people in this situation have gone through and still are going through. Similarly, in many years time you will have experienced perhaps even more dynamic times, if the present rate of change and sense of instability is anything to go by.

6.14 SUMMARY OF SKILLS USED AS A WAY TO MANAGE PROFESSIONAL ISSUES

The theme throughout this book has been that the beginner professional, working in most mental health settings, can contribute usefully to the care of many people suffering with mental illness using a range of rudimentary skills, techniques and ideas. These were explained, described and then demonstrated in a wide variety of clinical situations. Some of the situations were challenging even for a trained professional. The point being made, though, is that even many trained professionals use this relatively small number of clearly identified techniques, although with a greater level of sophistication and backed by considerably more experience than the beginner.

Chapter 6 has described a range of personal and professional issues and situations that many newly qualified nurses and some other professionals may encounter. The same range of clearly identified skills can be applied to many of these situations to manage them rather than just coping with them. Faced with any of the above, the effective professional mental health nurse would need to possess the following attributes (not in order of importance).

Skills used to manage professional issues ▶

- The ability to empathise
- The desire to be accepting and non-judgemental
- Honesty and integrity
- A genuine willingness to listen
- A high degree of self-awareness
- The ability to be approachable to a wide range of people
- An awareness of boundaries
- The ability to be intuitive

This sounds like a tall order but most people who work as mental health carers have these attributes, to a lesser or greater degree. Many of the above attributes appear in Chapter 1 as 'rudiments' and many are needed to effectively manage the situations described in Chapter 6. The skills are the same but they are used more selectively or more sensitively.

APPENDIX A
MEASURING THE PATIENT'S/CLIENT'S EXPERIENCE

USING A DIARY

Nathan's diary entry. Wednesday – 'Had a phone call from my sister this afternoon. Felt really down afterwards. I don't know why. She always has that effect on me. I remember when we were little she always used to bully me and get me into trouble. Perhaps that's the reason.

Nathan and his named nurse meet.

Nurse. So how did you get on with your diary last week?
Nathan. Nothing much happened at all. I had a call from my sister.
Nurse. So what did she say?
Nathan. It's not what she said, it's how she said it. She always seems to humiliate me somehow. I put it down in my diary, how she bullied me when we were kids.
Nurse. How did it feel when you wrote that?
Nathan. I couldn't believe how angry I felt. It's over 20 years ago!

USING A SCALE

Nurse. So on a scale of 1 to 10, where 1 is calm and 10 is really angry, how angry did you feel when you wrote that down?
Nathan. I'd say about 9.
Nurse. It's still very powerful then?
Nathan. Yes I can't believe it, I thought I'd dealt with all that stuff.
Nurse. How do you feel *now* on the same scale?
Nathan. About 6, but I can feel it getting worse again.

(See also Watkins 2001, p. 92.)

USING A PIE CHART

Nurse. Look at this piece of paper (draws a rough circle)
If this circle represents all your significant relationships, how much of it is taken up with your sister.
Nathan. Not much really. Most of it is taken up by my children. About this much (draws a segment). Then there's Lois – she's great with me! (draws another segment). Then of course my Dad (draws another segment)
Nurse. So there's not much room left for your sister is there?
Nathan. No. So why does she still get to me so much? She looks almost squashed out of this circle.
Nurse. Do you think she might feel like that?
Nathan. I'd never thought of it like that.

Pie chart showing Nathan's relationships sketched by the nurse

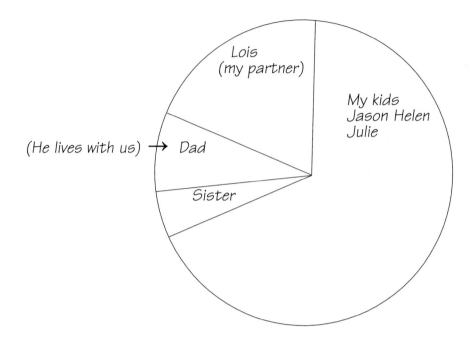

USING A CONTINUUM

Nurse. So what's good about your sister being squashed out of your circle and what's bad about it?

Nathan. What's good is that she's getting a taste of her own medicine. Now she knows how it feels to be left out. That's what she used to do to me.

Nurse. What's bad about it?

Nathan. I feel like I'm playing silly games. It doesn't make me feel good about me.

APPENDIX B
STAGES OF EGAN'S MODEL OF HELPING

(This also demonstrates how the stages need not necessarily be worked through in order.)

Stage 1: Telling the story

Nurse. So what were the events leading up to you being admitted yesterday, Beryl?

Beryl. Well I started feeling a bit down just after Christmas again. It's when I lost Philip in that accident. He just went out to play on his new bike. If only we'd not got him a bike!

Nurse. What do you think triggered it off this time – you've suffered like this before, haven't you?

Beryl. He would have been 18 this Christmas. It just seemed to hit me a lot harder this year. Everybody else seems to be celebrating and I just want to hide. Nobody understands.

Nurse. Does anybody know?

Beryl. I never talk about him. I've no-one to tell anyway since Joe went. The kids never mention him, so I just shut up about it.

Stage 2: Exploring the options

Nurse. How do you think you could manage this so you don't need to keep coming into hospital each time?

Beryl. I don't know. The kids won't talk about it. It's like he never existed.

Nurse. Have you ever tried mentioning him to your daughters?

Beryl. I daren't. They'd tell me not to be so stupid. They'd say 'Just forget him, Mum'.

Nurse. What do think about mentioning Philip to your daughter when she comes in tonight?

Beryl. No, I don't think so. I know you're trying to help.

Nurse. Well, it might be worth thinking about. You could be surprised. She might not tell you to just forget him. If you don't feel up to that, what else could you try?

Beryl. I'd quite like to talk to the vicar, perhaps?

Nurse. What stops you doing that?

Beryl. He always seems too busy.

Stage 3: Try them out/evaluate

A few days later.

Nurse. How are you this morning Beryl?

Beryl. I slept a bit better last night.

Nurse. How come?

Beryl. I phoned the vicar last night. He's coming to see me this afternoon. I told him what we talked about. He seemed to understand about Phil. I still don't think I can talk to my kids, though.

Nurse. Well, let's see how you feel after you've spoken to the vicar.

Stage 1: More telling the story

Beryl. I'm a bit nervous about seeing the vicar. I used to go to church a lot, every Sunday. Then when Joe left I stopped going. It all seemed pointless. I lost touch with a lot of people then.

Nurse. So in a way you've become quite isolated since you stopped going to church?

Beryl. I suppose so. I hadn't really thought about it much.

Stage 2: Exploring more options

Nurse. Can you think of any ways of getting people around you again? It seemed to help you before Joe went.

Beryl. I couldn't go to church again. I'd be on my own, I don't know anybody.

Nurse. How about asking the vicar how you can manage that?

Beryl. Ooh, I'm not sure.

Nurse. Any other ideas?

Beryl. Mrs Carr keeps pestering me to go to bingo, but it's not my thing.

Nurse. What is your thing?

Stage 1: More telling the story

Beryl. Well when me and Joe were together we used to go for long walks with Philip in the pram. I was really happy then.

APPENDIX C
HELP ORGANISATIONS AND NURSING UNIONS

Citizen's Advice Bureau. Website www.nacab.org.uk/

National Union of Students. Tel. 0207 272 8900; website www.nus.org.uk

NHS Direct. Tel. 0845 4647; website www.nhsdirect.nhs.uk

Parentline. Tel. 0808 800 2222; website www.parentlineplus.org.uk

RCN Counselling. Comprehensive website, need membership to enter. Telephone or face to face counselling service for members. Tel. 0845 769 7064; website accessible via 'RCN Counselling'.

Relate. Helpline 0845 130 4010; website www.relate.org.uk; e-mail enquiries@relate.org.uk

Samaritans. Tel. 08457 909090 (UK); 1850 609090 (Republic of Ireland); website www.samaritans.org.uk; e-mail jo@samaritans.org

Unison. Britain's biggest trade union. Has 1.3 million members, largely from the public services. Tel. 0845 355 0845; website www.unisondirect.org.uk; e-mail direct@unison.co.uk

REFERENCES

Abramowitz, J. S. (2001) CBT for obsessive compulsive disorder: a review of the treatment literature. *Research and Social Work Practice*, **11**(3), 357–372.

Adler, R. and Towne, N. (1999) *Looking Out, Looking In*, 9th edn, Harcourt Brace, Fort Worth, TX.

Aguilera, D. C. (1994) *Crisis Intervention: Theory and Methodology*, (7th edn), C. V. Mosby, St Louis, MO.

Altschuler, J. (1997) *Working with Chronic Illness*, Palgrave, Basingstoke.

American Psychiatric Association (1994) *DSM IV*, 4th edn, American Psychiatric Association, Washington, DC.

Annis, L. V. and Baker, C. A. (1986) A psychiatrist's murder in a mental hospital. *Hospital and Community Psychiatry*, **37**(5), 505–506.

Armson, S. (2003) Saving lives. *Mental Health Today*, **April**, 14–15.

Armstrong, L. and Wright, A. M. (2002) Communication in day care: talking, writing, networks. *Journal of Dementia Care*, **10**(6), 28–29.

Arnold, E. and Boggs, K. (2003) *Interpersonal Relationships*, 4th edn, W. B. Saunders, St Louis, MO.

Asai, A. (1995) Should physicians tell patients the truth? *Western Journal of Medicine*, **163**(1), 36–39.

Atkinson, R. L., Atkinson, R. C., Smith, E. E., Bem, D. J. and Nolen-Hoeksema, S. (1996) *Hilgard's Introduction to Psychology*, 12th edn, Harcourt Brace, Fort Worth, TX.

Barker, P. (1999) *The Philosophy and Practice of Psychiatric Nursing*, Churchill Livingstone, Edinburgh.

Barker, P. (2000) The philosophy of empowerment. *Mental Health Nursing*, **20**(9), 8–12.

Barker, P. (2003) Putting acute care in its place. *Mental Health Nursing*, **23**(1), 12–15.

Barker, P., Campbell, P. and Davidson, B. (eds) (2000) *From the Ashes of Experience*, Whurr, London.

Barraclough, C. (2003) A knife above the heart. *Mental Health Nursing*, **23**(4), 18–19.

Barry, P. D. (1998) *Mental Health and Mental Illness*, J. B. Lippincott, Philadelphia, PA.

Bates, P. (2002) Anyone who has a life. *Mental Health Today*, **May**, 21–24.

Baxter, E. (1992) Assaults by patients: the experiences and attitudes of psychiatric hospital nurses. *Australian and New Zealand Journal of Psychiatry*, **26**(4), 567–573.

Beer, D., Pereira, S. and Paton, C. (2001) *Psychiatric Intensive Care*, Greenwich Medical, Chatham.

Bergman, B. (1991) Suicide by battered wives. *Acta Psychiatrica Scandinavica*, **83**, 380–384.

Berne, E. (1975) *Games People Play*, Penguin, Harmondsworth.

Blackburn, I. M. and Davidson, K. M. (1990) *Cognitive Therapy for Depression and Anxiety. a Practitioner's Guide*, Blackwell Scientific, Oxford

Bloye, D. and Davies, S. (1999) *Psychiatry*. Mosby, London.

Borrill, J. (2000) Listening to dementia. *Mental Health Nursing*, **20**(1), 23.

Bradshaw, T. (2000) Psychosocial interventions and COPE. *Mental Health Nursing*, **20**(8), 10–14.

Bradshaw, T. and Haddock, G. (1998) Is befriending by trained volunteers of value to people suffering from long term mental illness? *Journal of Advanced Nursing*, **27**(4), 713–720.

Brooking, J., Ritter, S. and Thomas, B. (eds) (1992) *A Textbook of Psychiatric and Mental Health Nursing*, Churchill Livingstone, Edinburgh

Burnard, P. (1992) *Communicate!* Edward Arnold, London.

Burnard, P. (2003) Ordinary chat and therapeutic conversation: phatic communication and mental health nursing. *Journal of Psychiatric and Mental Health Nursing*, **10**(6), 678–682.

Bywaters, P. and Rolfe, A. (2002) Self help or self harm? *Mental Health Today*, **Nov**, 20–23.

Cardell, R., and Horton-Deutsch, S. (1994) A model for assessment of inpatient suicide potential. *Archives of Psychiatric Nursing*, **8**(6), 366–372.

Carson, V. B. (2000) *Mental Health Nursing*, 2nd edn, W. B. Saunders, Philadelphia, PA.

Casement, P. (1994) *On Learning From the Patient*, Routledge, London.

Charlton, B. (2000) *Psychiatry and the Human Condition*, Radcliffe Medical Press, Abingdon.

Christensen, H. (2003) Adjunctive cognitive therapy is more effective but more costly than standard clinical management for relapse prevention in depression. *Evidence Based Mental Health*, **6**(3), 85.

Clark, D. (1992) Understanding the development of the concepts of suicide through the use of early memory technique, *Death Studies*, **16**(4), 299–316.

Clarke, L. (1999) *Challenging Ideas in Psychiatric Nursing*, Routledge, London.

Coombs, R. (1996) From carers to custodians. Ethical dilemmas for community psychiatric nurse in the supervision of patients under the MHA 1983. *Nursing Times*, **92**(42), 19.

Concise Oxford Dictionary (1996) *Oxford English Dictionary* (eds J. Pearsall and B. Trumble), Oxford University Press, Oxford.

Crepaz-Kreay, D. (2003) Different but equal. *Mental Health Today*, **March**, 30–32.

Cutillo-Schmitter, T. (1996) Managing ambiguous loss in dementia and terminal illness. *Journal of Gerontological Nursing*, **22**(5), 32–39.

Dace, E. (2003) Diatribe. *Mental Health Today*, **June**, 37.

Department of Health (1992) *The Health of the Nation: a Strategy for Health in England*, HMSO, London.

Department of Health (2002a) *Adult Acute In-patient Care Provision*. Stationery Office, London.

Department of Health (2002b) *Journey to Recovery – the Government's Vision for Mental Health Care*. Stationery Office, London.

Department of Health (2003) *Statistics from Register of Drug Misuse Database in England 2000/01*, available on-line at www.doh.gov.uk/drugs/.

Donati, F. (1989) A psychodynamic observer in a chronic psychiatric ward. *British Journal of Psychotherapy*, **5**(3), 317–329.

Doyle, M. (1996) Assessing risk of violence from clients. *Mental Health Nursing*, **16**(3), 20–23.

Egan, G. (2002) *The Skilled Helper*, 7th edn, Brooks/Cole, Pacific Grove, CA.

Embling, S. (2002) The effectiveness of cognitive behavioural therapy in depression. *Nursing Standard*, **17**(14/15), 33–41.

Estoff, S. (1981) Psychiatric deinstitutionalisation: a sociocultural analysis. *Journal of Social Issues*, **37**(3), 116–132.

Evans, A. M. (1995) Philosophy of nursing: future directions. *Australian and New Zealand Journal of Mental Health Nursing*, **4**(1), 14–21.

Firn, S. (1995) Hobson's choice. *Nursing Times*, **91**(10), 56.

Fitzimons, S. (2002) Empowerment and its implications for clinical practice in mental health: a review. *Journal of Mental Health*, **11**(5), 481–99.

Forster, S. (ed.) (1997) *The A–Z of Community Mental Health Practice*, Stanley Thornes, Cheltenham.

Fredman, S. J., Fava, M., Kienke, A. S. *et al.* (2000) Partial response, nonresponse, and relapse with selective serotonin reuptake inhibitors in major depression: a survey of current 'next-step' practices. *Journal of Clinical Psychiatry*, **61**(6), 403–408.

Gelder, M., Mayou, R. and Geddes, J. (1999) *Psychiatry*, 2nd edn, Oxford University Press, Oxford.

Gibson, M. (1991) *Order From Chaos*, Venture Press, Birmingham.

Gillam, T. (2002) *Reflections on Community Psychiatric Nursing*, Routledge, London.

Gournay, K. (2003) Schizophrenia and NICE: another view. *Mental Health Nursing*, **23**(4), 14–15.

Gumley, A., O'Grady, M. and McNay, L. (2003) Early intervention for relapse in schizophrenia: results of a 12 month randomized controlled trial of cognitive behaviour therapy. *Psychological Medicine*, **33**(3), 412–431.

Hawton, K. (2001) The influence of the economic and social environment on deliberate self harm and suicide: an ecological and person based study. *Psychiatric Medicine*, **31**(5), 827–836.

Heron, J. (2001) *Helping the Client*, 5th edn, Sage Publications, London.

Hochberger, J. M. (1992) A discharge group for chronically mentally ill: easing the way. *Journal of Psychosocial Nursing and Mental Health Services*, **30**(4), 25–27.

Hopkins, C. and Walsey, S. (2002) Intervening safely in a crisis. *Mental Health Nursing*, **22**(4), 18–21.

Jackson, S. (1998) The gift of time from the friendly professional. *Nursing Standard*, **12**(51), 31–33.

Jacobson, J. and Jacobson, A. (1996) *Psychiatric Secrets*, Hanley & Belfus, Philadelphia, PA.

Johnstone, L. (2000) *Users and Abusers of Psychiatry*, Routledge, London.

Jones, A. (2002) Targeting suicide. *Mental Health Nursing*, **22**(6), 3.

Kane, J. M. (1999) Primary care psychiatry and schizophrenia: challenges and opportunities. *Primary Care Psychiatry*, **5**(4), 125–131.

Kaye, C. and Lingiah, T. (2000) *Race, Culture and Ethnicity in Secure Psychiatric Practice*, Jessica Kingsley, London.

Keene, J. (2001) *Complex Needs*, Blackwell, London.

Kuhn, D. and Verity, J. (2002) Putdowns and uplifts: signs of good or poor dementia care. *Journal of Dementia Care*, **10**(5), 26–28.

Lago, C. (1997) *Race, Culture and Counselling*, Open University Press, Buckingham.

Laurance. J. (2003) Pure madness: how fear drives the mental health system. Routledge, London.

Lego, S. (1996) *Psychiatric Nursing*, 2nd edn, J. B. Lippincott, Philadelphia, PA.

Libberton, P. (2000) Getting your ACT together. *Mental Health Nursing*, **20**(3), 14–17.

Lysaker, P. and Bell, M. (1995) Working and meaning: disturbance of volition and vocational dysfunction in schizophrenia. *Psychiatry*, **58**(4), 392–400.

McCarty, P. (1992) RNs use cues to predict violence. *American Nurse*, **24**(4), 6–9.

McGovern, M. and Whitcher, S. (1994) *Altschul's Psychiatric and Mental Health Nursing*, 7th edn. Baillière Tindall, London.

McHale, J., Tingle, J. and Peysner, J. (1998) *Law and Nursing*, 2nd edn, Butterworth-Heinemann, Oxford.

McLeod, J. (1998) *An Introduction to Counselling*, 2nd edn, Open University Press, Buckingham.

McLeod, J. (2003) *An Introduction to Counselling*, 3rd edn, Open University Press, Buckingham.

McSee, G. (1985) 'Hearing' non verbal cues in controlling aggressive patients. *Emotional First Aid: A Journal of Crisis Intervention*, **2**(3) 47–53.

Malone, B. (2003) *RCN Bulletin 77*, Royal College of Nursing, Harrow.

May, D. L. (1995) Patients' perceptions of self induced water intoxication. *Archives of Psychiatric Nursing*, **9**(5) 295–304.

Meadows, G. N. (2003) Overcoming barriers to reintegration of patients with schizophrenia: developing a best practice model for discharge from specialist care. *Medical Journal of Australia*, **178**(Suppl.), S53–S56.

Morrison, P. (1996) Patient satisfaction in a forensic unit. *Journal of Mental Health*, **5**(4) 369–377.

Moyle, W. (2002) Living with loss: dementia and the family care giver. *Australian Journal of Advanced Nursing*, **19**(3), 25–31.

Murdach, A. D. (1993) Working with potentially assaultive clients. *Health and Social Work*, **18**(4), 307–312.

Myers, D. G. (1993) *The Pursuit of Happiness*, Aquarian Press, London.

Nelson Jones, R. (1997) *The Theory and Practice of Counselling*, 2nd edn, Cassell, London.

Nelson Jones R (2002) *Essential Counselling and Therapy Skills: The Skilled Client Model*, Sage, London.

Newbigging, K. (2002) Not so easy. *Mental Health Today*, **October**, 12–13.

Newell, R. and Gournay, K. (2000) *Mental Health Nursing: an Evidence Based Approach*, Churchill Livingstone, Edinburgh.

Nhiwatiwa, F. G. (2003) The effects of single session education in reducing symptoms of distress following patient assault in nurses working in medium secure settings. *Journal of Psychiatric and Mental Health Nursing*, **10**(5), 561–568.

Nierenberg, A. A. (2001) Current perspectives on the diagnosis and treatment of major depressive disorder. *American Journal of Managed Healthcare*, **7**(11), 356–366.

NMC (2002) *Code of Conduct*, Nursing and Midwifery Council, London.

Norman, I. and Redfern, S. (1997) *Mental Health Care for Elderly People*, Churchill Livingstone, Edinburgh.

O'Brien, P., Kennedy, W. and Ballard, K. (1999) *Psychiatric Nursing*, McGraw Hill, New York.

Oei, P. S. (1999) The efficacy of cognitive processes of cognitive behaviour therapy in the treatment of panic disorder with agoraphobia. *Behavioural and Cognitive Psychotherapy*, **27**(1), 63–68.

O'Kane, P. and McKenna, B. (2002) Five a side makes the difference. *Mental Health Nursing*, **22**(5), 6–9.

Olds, J. (1995) The care of patients with dementia in general wards. *Professional Nurse*, **10**(7), 430–431.

Opbrock, A. (2002) Emotional blunting associated with SSRI. *International Journal of Neuropsychopharmacology*, **5**(2), 147–151.

Parker, G. and Roy, K. (2001) Assessing the comparative effectiveness of anti depressant therapies. *Journal of Clinical Psychiatry*, **62**(2), 117–125.

Polemeni-Walker, I. and Wilson, K. G. (1992) Reasons for participating in occupational therapy groups: perceptions of psychiatric in-patients and occupational therapists. *Canadian Journal of Occupational Therapy*, **59**(5), 240–247.

Prabhakaran, P. (2002) What are older people's experience of their antidepressants? *Journal of Affective Disorders*, **70**(3), 319–322.

Reed, A. (1998) Manufacturing a human drama from a psychiatric crisis: crisis intervention, family therapy and the work of R. D. Scott. *Journal of Psychiatric and Mental Health Nursing*, **5**(5), 387–392.

Rogers, C. R. (1951) *Client Centred Therapy*, Houghton Mifflin, Boston, MA.

Roper, N., Logan, W. W. and Tierney, A. J. (2000) *The Roper–Logan–Tierney Model of Nursing*, Churchill Livingstone, Edinburgh.

Royal College of Nursing (2003) *RCN Bulletin* 76, 1.

Royal College of Psychiatrists (2002) *Changing Minds*. Available on-line at: http://www.rcpsych.ac.uk/campaigns/cminds/printed_materials.htm.

Sammut, A. (2003) Developing an appropriate response to emotional pain. *Journal of Dementia Care*, **11**(2), 23–25.

Sathyamoorthy, G. (2001) Assessing cultural sensitivity. *Mental Health Today*, Sept, 16–19.

Simpson, K. (2002) Anorexia and culture. *Journal of Psychiatric and Mental Health Nursing*, **9**(1), 65–73.

Spender, Q., Salt, N., Dawkins, J., Kendrick, T. and Hill, P. (2001) *Child Mental Health in Primary Care*, Radcliffe Medical, Abingdon.

Stuart, G. and Laraia, M. (2001) *Principles and Practice of Psychiatric Nursing*, Mosby, St Louis, MO.

Suhail, K. (2002) Effect of culture and environment on the phenomenology of delusion and hallucinations. *International Journal of Social Psychiatry*, **48**(2), 126–138.

Thomas, B., Hardy, S. and Cutting, P. (1997) *Stuart and Sundeen's Mental Health Practice*, Mosby, London.

Thompson, S. (1999) The Internet and its potential influence on suicide. *Psychiatric Bulletin*, **23**(8) 449–451.

Thompson, I. (2000) Mental health and spiritual care. *Nursing Standard*, **17**(9), 33–38.

Thompson, T. and Mathias, P. (1994) *Lyttle's Mental Health and Disorder*, 2nd edn, Baillière Tindall, London.

Thorne, B. (2002) *The Mystical Power of Person Centred Therapy*, Whurr, London.

Tober, G. (1994) Drug taking in a northern city. *Accident and Emergency Nursing*, **2**(2), 70–78.

Turkington, D. (2002) Effectiveness of a brief cognitive behavioural therapy intervention in the treatment of schizophrenia. *British Journal of Psychiatry*, **180**(6), 523–527.

Turnbull, Q., Wolf, A. M. and Holroyd, S. (2003) Attitudes of elderly subjects toward truth telling for the diagnosis of Alzheimer's disease. *Journal of Geriatric Psychiatry and Neurology*, **16**(2) 90–93.

Van Os, J. (2003) Can the social environment cause schizophrenia? *British Journal of Psychiatry*, **182**, 291–292.

Varcarolis, E. (1998) *Foundations of Psychiatric/Mental Health Nursing*, W. B. Saunders, Philadelphia, PA.

Varcarolis, E. (2000) *Psychiatric Nursing Clinical Guide*, W. B. Saunders, Philadelphia, PA.

Veeramah, V. (2002) The benefits of using clinical supervision. *Mental Health Nursing*, **22**(1), 18–23.

Wareing, L. A. and Assey, J. (2001) Sense and sensitivity. *Mental Health Today*, **November**, 25–28.

Warner, L. and Nicholls, V. (2000) Spirit of understanding. *Mental Health Nursing*, **March**, 30–32.

Watkins, P. (2001) *Mental Health Nursing. The Art of Compassionate Care*, Butterworth-Heinemann, Oxford.

Wattis, J. P. (1994) Correlation between hospital anxiety depression (HAD) scale and other measures of anxiety and depression in geriatric inpatients. *International Journal of Geriatric Psychiatry*, **9**(1) 61–63.

Watts, A. (1987) *The Way of Liberation*, John Weatherill, New York.

Whittington, R. (1992) Staff strain and social support in a psychiatric hospital following assault by a patient. *Journal of Advanced Nursing*, **17**(4) 480–486.

Whittington, D. and McLaughlin, C. (2000) Finding time for patients: an exploration of nurses' time allocation in an acute psychiatric setting. *Journal of Psychiatric and Mental Health Nursing*, **7**(3), 259–268.

Williamson, T. (2003) Enough is good enough. *Mental Health Today*, **April**, 24–27.

World Health Organization (1992) *International Classification of Diseases*, 10th edn. Geneva, WHO.

Wright, H. and Giddey, M. (1993) *Mental Health Nursing*, Chapman & Hall, London.

Further reading

Chaloner, C. and Coffey, M., eds (2000) *Forensic Mental Health Nursing: Current Approaches*, Blackwell, Oxford.

Einstein, P. (2002) *Intuition, The Path to Inner Wisdom*, Vega, London.

Hope, A. (2000) Helping Mary. *Mental Health Nursing*, **20**(4), 18–21.

James, A. (2003) Phil Barker. *Openmind*, **119**, 9.

Jones, A. (2002) DBT and treating personality disorder. *Mental Health Nursing*, **22**(2), 6–9.

Lyttle, J. (1986) *Mental Disorder: Its Care and Treatment*, Baillière Tindall, London.

Reeves, T. (2003) Cognitive therapy and panic attacks. *Mental Health Nursing*, **23**(1), 16–19.

INDEX